NO EXCUSES
FITNESS

NO EXCUSES FITNESS

*The 30-Day Plan to Tone Your Body
and Supercharge Your Health*

DONOVAN GREEN
with
RICHARD McGILL MURPHY

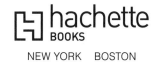
hachette
BOOKS

NEW YORK   BOSTON

Copyright © 2015 by Donovan Green
Photographs by Eddie Berman

Hachette Books
Hachette Book Group
1290 Avenue of the Americas
New York, NY 10104

www.HachetteBookGroup.com

Printed in the United States of America

RRD-C

First edition: April 2015
10 9 8 7 6 5 4 3 2 1

Hachette Books is a division of Hachette Book Group, Inc.
The Hachette Books name and logo are trademarks of Hachette Book Group, Inc.

The publisher is not responsible for websites (or their content) that are not owned by the publisher.

Library of Congress Cataloging-in-Publication Data has been applied for.

CONTENTS

PREFACE

By Lisa Oz

Chance encounters can change your life. Years ago I practiced martial arts at a dojo near my home in New Jersey. I noticed that a tall, very fit man would show up often to watch the class I was in. He was always happy, always smiling, and always in incredible shape. I was curious about him, so after a couple of weeks I introduced myself and we got to talking.

He told me that his name was Donovan Green, from Jamaica by way of the South Bronx. He worked as a fitness coach and came to our dojo to support his beautiful wife Ayana, a martial artist who often trained in my class. I loved Donovan's energy (plus I wanted to know how he stayed so ripped), so I asked him to train me.

I thought we would use the latest and greatest exercise gear available, and I started to list all the possibilities. Donovan nodded politely, and then proceeded to put me through one of the most fun, challenging workouts I had ever experienced.

We didn't use a single piece of equipment. Instead, Donovan showed me how to build cardiovascular endurance and muscular strength using nothing more than the resistance of my own body. After that, Donovan and I started training together regularly. He also trained my husband and appeared as a guest on *The Dr. Oz Show*.

I believe Donovan has an important message to share with the world, which is why I'm so happy that he has written this book. Donovan understands that there's much more to fitness than simply working out. True fitness is about lifestyle transformation. It requires sound nutrition, mental strength, and emotional balance. Ultimately, it demands spiritual serenity. Donovan's No Excuses program helped me build fitness on all these fronts, and it can help you too. I think the world would be a better place if everyone in it read this book.

PROLOGUE

Training Shoshana

Shoshana Smith weighed about 300 pounds when she first walked into my gym on Prospect Avenue in the South Bronx. With a personality to match her figure, she sashayed up to the front desk and demanded the best trainer in the building. I sat down with Shoshana and asked a few questions, just to get to know her a little better. I learned that she was unemployed and raising her two young children on her own. She hoped to improve her financial situation by becoming a court officer. The problem was that she needed to lose 100 pounds to be eligible for the force.

Shoshana had already washed out of many fitness and weight-loss programs, mostly because she lost confidence in herself. But now she had a real deadline. The next court officer exam was a year away, so she had 52 weeks to lose one-third of her body weight, or she wouldn't even be eligible to take it. As an experienced fitness coach I knew Shoshana's goal was difficult but achievable, and I could tell she was ready for the journey no matter what. She was living on personal savings and government assistance at the time, so I cut her a deal on the training fees and we started working out almost immediately. There was no time to waste.

Shoshana was the perfect candidate to join my No Excuses program, a holistic health plan based on a tripod of smart nutrition, intense mental training, and targeted physical exercise. I put her on a strict diet of 1,500 calories a day and launched her on my total-body-workout regimen, which combines yoga, Pilates, weights, and mixed martial arts. We worked out for 45 minutes a day, 5 days a week, varying the workout every day so that Shoshana was constantly challenged and never bored. Within 4 months she had dropped 30 pounds.

After 6 months on the program, even though she was sticking to her diet and exercise regime and despite all her progress, Shoshana became impatient with the rate at which she was losing weight. Never a wallflower, she got right up in my face at the gym and announced that she didn't feel that the No Excuses program was working for her anymore.

Soon thereafter, Shoshana bought $200 worth of fat-burning pills. She brought the box containing her new pills to the gym and showed them to me, thinking that I would approve. I asked her to put the pills into my hand. Then I developed a mysterious "hand tremor" and spilled them all out on the floor. Oops! Suddenly I faced an enraged client with crazy martial arts skills that I'd taught her. Fighting an instinctive temptation to flee, I explained that diet pills are dangerous because they can increase your blood pressure and heighten your risk of heart disease. I told Shoshana that we were going to take her weight off the right way—the No Excuses way. Luckily for me she calmed down, and we started training again.

What I discovered that day was that Shoshana was focusing way too much on her bathroom scale. She weighed herself every day, and every day she'd get depressed about the results. I told her that scale was the devil and made her promise that she would weigh herself only once a month. Instead we focused on her body-fat percentage and on her measurements: waist, hips, bust, and thighs. Meanwhile she worked on seeing the connection between her mind and her body more clearly.

As the weeks went by, the numbers all dropped, and Shoshana's confidence increased. Once she opened her mind to change, she found balance, endurance, speed, power, and, ultimately, strength. And even though she wasn't weighing herself very often, her weight dropped steadily as well. After another 6 months of hard work and smart nutrition, Shoshana had made huge strides in the No Excuses program. She achieved her weight-loss goal and then some. Her weight dropped to 180 pounds without drugs or surgery, while her blood pressure went from dangerously high to normal.

Shoshana got so excited about fitness that she decided to forget about becoming a court officer. Instead she chose to manage my gym and go on to a successful career as a personal trainer. Four years later we're still good friends, and I'm happy to report that she has kept the weight off.

Remember, Shoshana started her fitness journey as an overweight, unemployed single mom. Bottom line: By following the No Excuses program and learning to let go of what wasn't working, Shoshana Smith turned her life around and achieved her fitness and life goals.

CHAPTER 1

No Excuses!

You probably have a pretty good idea about what it takes to shed unwanted pounds, which is to eat right and stay active. But if you're reading this, you must still need some help. Before we start this journey, you need to decide if you are ready to do what it takes to succeed.

I'm Donovan Green, personal trainer to Dr. Mehmet Oz, the TV personality, author, and health authority. As a fitness coach, motivational speaker, and frequent guest on *The Dr. Oz Show*, I've helped thousands of folks achieve their health and fitness goals. I wrote this book because I want to share my proven steps to physical and mental fitness with the world.

This book lays out a 30-day program designed to move anyone into a more active, healthy, and emotionally positive lifestyle. The program rests on three pillars—exercise, food, and attitude—and it requires a commitment. Every day you'll spend 20 minutes working out. You'll prepare healthy, delicious meals inspired by my Caribbean heritage. And you'll do mental exercises that will strengthen your mind and spirit to meet all the challenges that life can throw at you.

For the next 30 days, I am going to push you like you've never been pushed before. My job is to be your best trainer, not your best friend. I will not accept excuses. I will never allow you to tell yourself that you can't or you won't. That is fear trying to show its nasty face. Fear makes people crazy and drives them to their own destruction. Fear lurks in the shadows waiting quietly to take you out, and I don't mean for a stroll in the park. Fear is the mother of excuses, and excuses are the mother of failure.

Here's the first and most important step to achieving your fitness goals: *Stop making excuses!* Over the years I've heard every excuse in the book for not working out and eating right. *I chowed that entire chocolate cheesecake because my boss gave me a hard time at work yesterday. I haven't exercised in a year because I'm trying to pass the bar. I eat fast food every day because I don't have time to cook. I lost my job, so I can't afford to go to the gym. I'm gainfully employed, but I still can't go to the gym because my spouse left me, my kid is flunking out of school, and my cat ate a prize cockatoo that belonged to my neighbor, who now hates me. Did I mention that my knee hurts?*

Though I sympathize when people go through hard times, I don't accept adversity as an excuse to quit. I started my fitness journey as an overweight immigrant kid from Kingston, Jamaica. Growing up poor in the South Bronx during the 1980s crack epidemic, I saw my share of adversity. There were plenty of times when I wanted to give up. But I didn't give up. Instead I learned how to power through obstacles by training my body and mind for success. Most important, I learned to stop blaming the world for my problems. I stopped making excuses. You can too.

You will not get a free pass here, so please forget about your issues for a moment and pay strict attention to what I am about to tell you. Any reason you give for not being able to get fit is just an excuse, no matter how convincing it may sound. If you have time to watch TV, eat at a restaurant, have sex, talk on the phone, or go to work, then you have time to commit to being healthy.

It's all about the attitude. Back when I first started training Dr. Oz, we used to work out at his house in New Jersey on Saturday mornings. In those days Dr. Oz wasn't the star he is today, although he had made a name for himself as a featured physician on *The Oprah Winfrey Show.* One day we were doing push-ups together, and Dr. Oz was struggling big-time. But he didn't give up. Instead he looked over at me and gasped, "Hey, Donovan, is that all you got?"

I've always been impressed by Dr. Oz's drive to succeed and by his total lack of ego. Although I'm still Dr. Oz's trainer, I've come to see him more as a big brother than as a client. We're both high-energy, we both like to inspire others, and we share the same holistic view of health and fitness. Fundamentally, we both understand the importance of taking full responsibility for our own success.

I am not very nice or understanding when it comes to excuses. All I want is the best for you and nothing less. I do not want to hear about how hard your life is. If you have knee problems, you can still move your arms. If you have shoulder problems, you can still move your legs. If you are sitting in a wheelchair, you can still contract your stomach. If you suffer from couch syndrome, you can simply get up and move.

I don't care how young, old, or out of shape you are. We all have to start somewhere.

I won't lie and say this is the easiest thing you will ever do. On the contrary, it's one of the hardest jobs you will ever undertake. Getting and staying fit—mentally and physically—is a life-changing event that requires diligence and the highest level of commitment. But if the commitment is great, the reward will be equally so.

LOSE THE EXCUSE

On a blank sheet of paper, write down your favorite excuses not to exercise or eat right: *I'm too busy, I'm too tired, I have a slow metabolism, etc.*—all the usual suspects. When your list is complete, get a black garbage bag and throw that piece of paper in the bag. You are now done with excuses! As you gain more control over your nutrition, your physical fitness, and your mental attitude, you'll find it easier to eliminate excuses from your life and the garbage bag will become a metaphor.

CAN MONEY BUY FITNESS?

You can find a million excuses not to exercise or eat right. Without question, the excuse I hear most often is "I don't have the money." You might expect richer people to be healthier. Affluent communities tend to have good air quality, low crime, ample public recreation facilities, and well-funded schools with strong physical education programs. It obviously takes money to join the most expensive fitness clubs, hire the best nutritionists and personal trainers, and pay for great medical care.

Yet there's no shortage of obesity among upper-income Americans. For example, black and Mexican American men with higher incomes are more likely to be obese than their less affluent peers, according to research by the Centers for Disease Control (CDC). And even though folks with more education tend to earn more money, the CDC found no significant relationship between obesity and education in men. (College-educated women, on the other hand, are less likely to be obese than women with less education.)

Obesity follows naturally in a society where hardworking, time-strapped citizens meet cheap and ubiquitous junk food. Americans have been working harder and harder in recent decades. In the manufacturing sector, for example, U.S. labor productivity accelerated in the decades after 1973, even while it slowed in other industrial countries, according to the Bureau of Labor Statistics. At the same time, middle-class incomes have stagnated and job security has declined, as anyone who lived through the Great Recession of 2007 to 2009 can attest.

Particularly in tough economic times, it's natural to put your job ahead of your health. High-paying jobs are generally no less demanding than low-paying jobs. It's true that financially blessed folks can take time off from work and not worry about making rent. Yet even prosperous Americans face the universal, nagging fear that they'll sink back to the bottom if they stop working.

From a health and fitness perspective, having too much money is almost as bad as having too little. What do I mean? Money can make you lazy. It allows you to feed any addiction you have, be it drugs, sex, alcohol, or food. I've met many wealthy folks who didn't care to exercise or eat a healthy diet. They were too comfortable enjoying the luxuries their incomes afforded them.

Life is very different in low-income communities like my old neighborhood in the Bronx. Back in the BX, work and money were both scarce. Folks didn't always know where the next meal was coming from, and as a result they tended to focus on survival rather than exercising or eating a healthy diet. Gym membership was prohibitively expensive for most. Particularly during the 1980s crack epidemic, working out outdoors wasn't the best idea because of the high probability of getting robbed, attacked, or caught in cross fire.

Healthy food is scarce in poor communities, so people tend to buy whatever food is cheap and available. That often means fast food with its dangerous levels of fat, salt, and refined sugar. Stress levels are also very high. Is it any surprise that obesity is rife in these communities, or that folks are dying every day from illnesses related to obesity?

That said, I'm living proof that poverty doesn't have to make you fat. So are all the people who trained at my gym in the South Bronx. Many of them could barely make rent, and yet they still managed to exercise and eat right. I used to run my own fitness program for inner-city schoolchildren. Many of these kids were not used to moving around. I gave them a fun, interactive workout: Who could do the most jumping jacks and squat thrusts? Who could punch their way fastest through a martial arts routine? Their parents used to tell me they'd never seen their kids move so much. I've also worked with a lot of elderly clients, teaching them simple rejuvenating moves like arm circles, toe touches, neck stretches, and so on.

Bottom line: It doesn't matter if you're rich or poor, young or old, black or white. Anybody can live a healthier life. You just have to make fitness your number one priority. It's all about developing the willingness—the No Excuses attitude—to make that happen.

CHANGE YOUR WAYS

It's time to break any bad habits that might be getting between you and your fitness goals. I'm not saying that's easy. If your morning routine includes coffee and doughnuts in front of the morning news, you may find it challenging to substitute a 3-mile run followed by a protein shake. If you're used to buying corn dogs and bacon cheeseburgers for lunch, it's going to take some effort to pack a healthy meal in a cooler every morning and bring it with you to work.

And yet changing your lifestyle can be very simple, once you learn to stop making excuses. Take a moment to examine your life. Look at the things you are doing that might not be so great for your health. Write those things down on paper, and make sure to be 100 percent honest with yourself. This is where progress begins.

Telling yourself the truth might sound easy, but it isn't. If you know you are lazy, don't make excuses by saying you are just tired from work or school. Look deeper into your past and remember how you lived when you didn't have to work so many hours. Did you move around a lot, or were you still sitting on that couch? If you answered "couch," you're lazy in my book. No excuses, no reasons, just lazy.

Once you've written down all of your bad habits truthfully, get ready to make some serious changes. Pick one bad habit off the list and tell yourself out loud: *I will no longer do this, because I deserve to live better.* If you found nothing wrong, there are two possibilities: Either you're perfect or you're fooling yourself. Only the universe is perfect, so option two must be correct. (Note to students: This method also works on standardized tests!)

Once you've identified your bad habits, you must announce your decision to a close friend, spouse, or relative. This will help keep you accountable. It's always a great idea to tell others about your mission to get healthy. You won't want to fail once you know that others are watching.

STEP BY STEP

Think about this for a second. When you want to go somewhere in your car, you don't just jump in and drive. Instead you follow a series of steps: opening the door, sitting down, putting on your seat belt, checking your mirrors, pushing the key into the ignition, and so on. No matter how expensive or fast the car is, you can't drive it without first taking those critical steps.

Lifestyle change works the same way. Don't make the mistake of thinking you can get healthy all in one shot. You have to take it slow and wean yourself from your bad habits.

We all have things that we can stop doing immediately. For example, I can stop being someone's friend at the snap of a finger. I can go forever without riding my motorcycle. (I really love my motorcycle.) But I find it much harder to maintain healthy diet choices. It takes daily effort. By and large I eat a healthy vegetarian diet, but sometimes I fall off the wagon and guzzle a bag of Oreos with my son. The point is that I always get right back on the wagon.

You are perfect only at making mistakes. After every mistake you must get back up, brush yourself off, and start again. Here's the good news: Changing your lifestyle won't just help you manage your weight. It will also help you achieve peak performance in every aspect of your life. Once you look and feel your best, you will always feel like you are in total control.

We all value our lives. Most of us would lie, cheat, and even kill if it was the only way to go on living. During my career as a fitness coach, I've seen many folks try to change their lifestyle after a doctor's diagnosis. They join gyms, make appointments with nutritionists, and get massages. Sometimes they even start going to church. But why wait for your doctor to tell you the bad news before you decide to do something about your health?

Stop disease from happening right now. Not tomorrow, *right now*! Do it while you have your health. Time is of the essence, so make it count. Any reason you give for not being able to make a life change is just an excuse, no matter how convincing it may sound. If you're going to make excuses, try to make them positive, pertaining to the reasons why you work out rather than why you don't. For example: *I work out because I need to be stronger. I eat a lot of vegetables because I hate being sick*. Let those be your excuses to not make excuses.

DON'T FEAR SUCCESS

I am convinced that most people fail because they are fearful of success. It's always easier to blame someone or something else for your downfall. Over the years I've met many talented people who settled for less rather than making the effort to push hard and fast in life. Why? Some felt they weren't good enough. Others couldn't stand to be told no. Still others didn't know where to start or felt comfortable in their current situation.

Well, I say, *hell no*! That is unacceptable. I want you to live like you never lived before. Get your butt out there and take chances. Look fear in the eye and knock it out of the box. If you dream about going back to school, then get up off the couch, call a school you like, inquire about the steps you need to take, and enroll. If you want to lose weight, then stop eating those darn cheese fries and drinking so much alcohol and toxic soda. That's a start, and we all have to start somewhere.

Are you afraid of failure? Don't be. All successful people have failed at some point in their lives. The difference is that they learned from their failures, got right back up, and fought again. This program is going to demand a lot from you, both physically and mentally. If you truly want to survive my program, I expect you to give me your all. You are going to have to lose the excuses and open your mind to a brand-new path.

As a matter of fact, you are going to have to break that peace treaty with yourself. I want you to go to *war*! You must learn how to defeat yourself on this battlefield called life. Put down the shield of insecurities that you've been hiding behind all these years. Pick up your mental sword and slice your way through everything that drags you down.

I do not believe in settling for anything. If you settle you will not reach your full potential and you will not be truly happy. There will always be a sense of doubt lurking through your mind because you did not fulfill your goals. You only went halfway. Well, what if you didn't stop at halfway? What would happen if you went all the way?

Many people take the road of least resistance because they are afraid of fighting the battle. They are also too busy living up to the expectations of others instead of living for themselves. I want you to take the road of resistance. This is the road that will show you who you really are. It separates the men from the boys and the women from the girls.

Every great achievement started as a dream. Where would we be if Martin Luther King Jr. had kept his dream to himself? If Benjamin Franklin had never flown his kite in a thunderstorm? What if Dr. Oz had never gone to medical school? There would be a lot more people buried right now.

The richest place in the world is the cemetery because people die every day along with their gifts and dreams. So don't be afraid to live. I want you to stop talking about all the things you'd like to do someday. Instead, start getting them done.

Are you with me so far? I hope so, because now is your time to shine. The spotlight is on you and no one else. I am going to equip you with the tools you need to survive this battle and come out triumphant. I'm going to lead you to water, but I can't make you drink. You must show the world that you have what it takes to win. Your failure or success will be determined solely by your choices and your actions.

WHAT YOU NEED TO SURVIVE THIS PROGRAM

We are all born with the natural ability to survive. If you want to know the art of survival, just watch the nearest baby. A baby will cry, scream, kick, and throw tantrums just to survive. This is how a baby communicates when it is hungry, sick, angry, or tired.

Just like a baby, you must put yourself first in order to survive this program. I will accept nothing less from you. There is no more room for excuses, reasons, or *I will do it later.*

Now let's talk about the work involved. Exercise plays a big role, but not as big as you might think. Don't misunderstand me: Exercise is extremely important for both physical and physiological purposes. That's why I'm in the gym at least 5 days per week, busting my butt and sweating like I just got caught breaking the law.

However, the fitness industry wants you to believe that exercise is the only way to lose weight. If this were true, all those people who run off to the gym to get their bodies in shape for summer would be uniformly ripped. You and I both know that's not the case. Going to the gym and busting your butt is not going to change your body if you don't also change your lifestyle.

That means eating properly and maintaining mental focus. You need to plan each day before it begins and follow your plan by the book. Maybe you think you don't have time to exercise or prepare your meals ahead of time. You might even think that's normal. Well, guess what! It *is* normal: Millions of Americans feel the same way. Which means you have a choice to make. Do you want to be in the normal category or do you want to be in the elite category?

What you answer will largely determine where you end up with this program and with your life. Excuses are just a fast way out. They are easy and free of charge. But what if the world were different? What if you could make only one excuse per year? How would your life be then?

I think you'd be in a much better place. Your level of honesty would be higher. Your bank account would be more stable. Your relationships would be stronger, and your health would probably be at its best. Of course, I'm not psychic, so maybe all those things are great for you now. But remember: Only the universe is perfect.

THE NO EXCUSE ZONE

As a fitness coach, I've heard every excuse in the book from clients who don't want to exercise and eat right. The only one I'll accept is death, certified by a coroner. If you want to get fit, you need to stop making excuses!

Client	Donovan
I'm too busy.	All I need is 30 minutes.
I can't afford it.	Your living room is free.
I have an injury.	We'll work around it. Fitness speeds recovery.
My kids get in the way.	Train with them!
I'm fine the way I am.	I love you too. Now, gimme some push-ups.
I have a slow metabolism.	That's about to change. Let's start with jumping jacks.
I'm too tired.	Exercise gives you energy. Get up and move!
I died last Tuesday.	Fair enough.

CHAPTER 2

The Wellness Tripod

No matter where you fall on the continuum from couch potato to Olympic athlete, fitness comes from a balanced regime of exercise, sound nutrition, and mental discipline. I call this the Wellness Tripod. I'm talking big-picture wellness, not the quick fix of helping you lose 50 pounds by next Saturday so you can wear that old prom dress to your high school reunion. If you follow my No Excuses program diligently, you can count on losing the first 10 pounds within 30 days, without deprivation or misery. And I'll give you the tools to sustain that success and keep the weight off. But at heart, I'm not that kind of numbers guy. I'm far more into seeing you fit into your clothes comfortably. I want to see you healthy and able to do all the things you'd like to do. In short, I want to help you live a long, high-quality life.

I designed the No Excuses program with overweight and sedentary folks especially in mind. These are people who may feel defeated, people who've tried to lose weight but have failed or given up. And there are a lot of you. Nearly 55 million adult Americans engage in no physical exercise whatsoever outside work, according to the United Health Foundation. Physical inactivity increases the risk of developing serious illnesses like cardiovascular disease, diabetes, and hypertension. It also correlates with social problems such as undereducation, violent crime, and poverty. Physical inactivity is estimated to cause nearly 200,000 deaths in this country every year, and about $24 billion in direct medical spending.

Here's the good news: You don't have to be a statistic. There's a much better way to live, and this program will show you how to do it. As a fitness coach, I'm about opening clients' minds to possibility and optimism. I will lead you to success. I became a fitness coach after practicing martial arts for many years. The martial arts taught me self-discipline, humility, and respect for myself and my peers. At the physical level, the martial arts have enhanced my body mechanics, positioning, flexibility, and speed. I've incorporated this sensibility into my total-body workouts, fusing mixed martial arts with circuit training. On a deeper level, I will teach you the importance of being present at all times, of taking control so you can live your life to the fullest.

I've designed my program to suit all fitness levels, from couch potato to black belt. It incorporates weight lifting and exercises from yoga, Pilates, and mixed martial arts into a single cross-training system. If you practice these specialized movements diligently, you'll achieve flexibility with stability, stability with endurance, endurance with speed, speed with power, and power with strength. In short, you'll be a complete athlete.

Every athlete knows that there's more to fitness than just working out. True fitness also requires smart nutrition and mental discipline. These are the three legs of the Wellness Tripod. Here's my promise to you: If you eliminate the word "excuse" from your vocabulary and follow the advice in this book consistently, you will maintain peak fitness for the rest of your life. Nothing and nobody can stand in your way.

WHY ARE AMERICANS SO HEAVY?

In recent years, obesity has emerged as a major topic in American public life. First Lady Michelle Obama has led a national conversation about the connection between obesity and poor nutrition, especially in inner-city "food deserts" like the Bronx neighborhood where I launched my career as a fitness coach and motivational speaker. I created my No Excuses program because I want to be part of the solution to this problem.

Simply put, Americans are too fat because we don't exercise enough and we put all kinds of toxic garbage into our bodies. These habits get formed early in life. The U.S. food and beverage industry spends about $2.5 billion a year on marketing programs for children and teenagers, according to the Federal Trade Commission, much of it devoted to selling junk food that has been deliberately engineered to be addictive.

The good news is that the obesity epidemic has sparked creative, hopeful responses throughout this country, designed to help people ditch the bad habits that drag them down and make them fat. In the Mississippi Delta, one of the poorest and least healthy regions in the United States, a pastor named Dr. Michael Minor attracted national attention by banning fried chicken at church potlucks and installing a walking track around the church perimeter. "You can see the difference," Minor told Reuters. "People are much better sized, way better. And once they get it off, they want to keep it off."

I can relate to Dr. Minor because I've had similar experiences running a community gym in the South Bronx, visiting New York City public schools to teach lower-income kids about fitness, training affluent clients in the Connecticut suburbs, leading wellness seminars throughout the Northeast, and connecting with national audiences via *The Dr. Oz Show*. I've found the same hunger for wellness in all these settings.

The time demands on our lives are often so overwhelming that we lose focus on ourselves. We devote ourselves to our jobs and our families. Fitness takes a backseat—if it's even in the car. There are also those who were born with more dominant fat cells than the average person. Some of these folks have tried everything possible but never lost the weight.

America is highly advanced in technology, which ironically has put us far behind when it comes to health and fitness. There is almost no need for us to use our brains or muscles to complete a chore. Then there's temptation, amplified by the power of modern marketing. The average child hears, views, and reads up to 10,000 ads about food a year, according to the American Academy of Pediatrics, most of them selling junk food. The typical American diet is heavy on cheeseburgers, French fries, fried chicken, and cola. How can we possibly not get the urge to eat that beautiful slice of chocolate cake covered with fudge, caramel, and hot chocolate syrup?

Americans are also busy people. We chow whatever's handy because we're always on the go. One of the most common excuses for not exercising is *I don't have enough time*. But if you have time to watch TV, eat in restaurants, hang out with your friends, and go to nightclubs, then you definitely have time to exercise and eat right.

IS FITNESS GENETIC?

Have you or someone you know ever committed to an exercise and nutrition program, only to find that your body still looked the same after a year? You've probably also met folks who manage to look great without taking much exercise or watching their diets. Doesn't that make you sick to your stomach? How does that even happen to them and not to you?

Let's start with your genes. Take a hard look at your parents, grandparents, uncles, aunts, and cousins. Are they more on the small or big side? Your genetic heritage does play a role in how your body looks. Some people are genetically programmed to be lean and muscular—others, not so much. Does that mean you can get in shape only if you have the right genes? Absolutely not. You will be able to achieve a great physique, but not necessarily the one you expected.

Take me, for example. I'm blessed with a great set of arm and chest muscles from my father's side. Thanks to my dad's genes, I also have toothpick-looking ankles and calf muscles. I got my beauty from my mother, of course. Anyway, no matter how much I train my legs, I seem to be stuck with the same ankles and calves.

I have been able to tone and strengthen my lower legs. I can squat 365 pounds with perfect form, leg press more than 900 pounds, and complete a full leg extension with the whole rack. So why don't my legs look like the Hulk's? Because I don't have the Hulk's genes—that's why. On the plus side, I'm not green and I don't have a violent temper. Over the years I've learned to accept my genetic limitations and be proud of the body that God gave me.

Your genes play a major role in your looks. For example, not everyone is designed to have six-pack abs. I know there are a lot of people who will disagree with me on this. And there's no question that anyone can build more abdominal definition by exercising and cutting body fat down to about 14 percent for women and 8 percent for men. But that still doesn't guarantee you a six-pack. Some folks are as skinny as twigs and have a one-pack. Should they lose more weight too? I would think not.

Female clients often ask me if they can get a bigger or smaller butt from exercising. My answer is always a big, bold *no*. Your genes largely determine the size of your behind. However, you will be able to get your butt in better shape by toning those rear muscles using exercises such as my Lose That Thut workout on page 137. That's the truth and nothing "butt" the truth.

RE-CREATE YOUR CIRCLE

Your circle of friends can make or break you. There may be someone in your circle who has bad intentions for you. Allow your friends to be your friends but not your influence, especially if the influence is negative. You don't need to skip your workout just because your buddy wants company at the movies. You don't need to accept that late-night drink or eat that cheeseburger dripping with extra ketchup just because your friends offered it.

You must be prepared to lose friends when you make significant changes in your life. Years ago, I lost friends when I committed to fitness and stopped going out to nightclubs every weekend. If you choose to do something positive with your life and your so-called friends try to put a stick in your wheel, you must simply let them go.

Re-create your circle; get rid of anyone who has been a hindrance in your life. I don't mean feed them rat poison or throw them off a cliff. I simply mean that you need to change your environment if it's holding you back. If you just got out of rehab for drug abuse, don't go hang out with your old drug buddies. If you do, you are setting yourself up for a relapse.

There are no exceptions to this rule. In the past you may have tried to please your friends just to avoid hurting their feelings. Well, maybe that was part of your problem! True friends will support you in your No Excuses efforts. But anybody who is going to aid and abet your excuse making—you don't need them in your life.

The good news is that you may not have to work too hard at this if you stay on your path. Friends often drift apart because their lifestyles no longer match. So those bad influences may be gone before you know it.

CHOOSE HEALTH

The choice is so simple when it comes to getting fit. You either do it or you don't. Even if you don't happen to feel like exercising, you do it anyway because the alternatives are so much worse. I personally love to exercise, but I hate vegetables. I still eat them, though, because I know how important they are to my health. I know my body needs the nutrients provided by vegetables, so I consume at least four servings per day. I'll eat my veggies steamed or raw. Sometimes I throw them into a blender and drink them down. No matter how I fix my veggies, I don't love eating them. I do it because my body is my home. Where would I live if I didn't have it?

Wake up and smell the fresh fruits and vegetables! You live in the jungle, which can be a very dangerous place. You must be strong and confident to escape people and things that can hurt you. This is the time for you to drop the entire BS syndrome in your life and step outside the box. I need you to think about *you* right now and no one else. Does that sound selfish? It should. It's not always a bad thing to be selfish. You have spent plenty of time living for your boss, your colleagues, your family, and your friends. In the long run your lifestyle change will benefit all these people. Right now it's all about you.

> "Time is free, but it's priceless. You can't own it, but you can use it. You can't keep it, but you can spend it. Once you've lost it you can never get it back."
> —Harvey Mackay

> ## FRIENDSHIP, DEFINED
>
> A real friend is someone who makes you a better person. At the very least, a friend doesn't stand in your way if you're trying to change for the better. Right now, I want you to make a list of people you consider to be friends. Ask yourself, do these people want what is best for me? If the answer is no, they probably don't belong on the list—or in your life.

TIME IS NOT ON YOUR SIDE

Though I believe in taking life one day at a time, I don't expect you to take your time with this program. I want you to simply take the plunge. Just jump right in and tell yourself you can do this. What if you don't know how to swim? I guess it's either sink or learn to swim, right? Life is hard, and only the fit survive. You have no time to waste.

I don't expect you to change overnight, but I do expect you to start changing overnight. I want you to be patient but also impatient. Start breaking those nasty habits as soon as possible. Think about it this way. You've spent your whole life taking your time. How far has it gotten you? I'm not telling you to jump out of bed and go for a 10-mile run if you've never done it before. What I am saying is get your butt out of bed and go for a run. How many times have you set a goal in your life, said *I have until this specific time to get there*, and then failed way before the deadline even arrived?

The reason why you failed is because *you took your time*. Chances are you also failed to plan. Once again: Time is not on your side. If you tell yourself that all you have is time, then you'll develop what I call the "what's the hurry?" syndrome. I want you to be in enough of a hurry to fully engage now and not tomorrow. The more time you believe you have, the more time you will lose.

My wife and I recently watched the movie *In Time*, starring Justin Timberlake. It's about a dystopic future in which people spend time instead of money. Everybody has a digital clock inserted into their forearms at birth. The clock doesn't budge until you hit twenty-five years of age, and then *boom!* It starts ticking. There is no money in this world. Instead you spend units of time for everything you need. The richest characters in the movie are the folks with the most time on their clocks. Physically, everyone in the film looks young and beautiful. But they all drop dead the moment their personal clocks click down to zero.

I loved *In Time* because it made so much sense. We all take time for granted, thinking we have a lot of it when in reality we don't. When your time is up, your time is up—end of story. Once again, I'm not saying you have to do everything all in one day. If you try, you will fail miserably. I simply want you to understand that you must act now or you will continue to lose opportunities to change.

Rome wasn't built in a day, but it would never have been built at all if some Romans hadn't climbed off their couches and gotten started. Don't make the mistake of sitting on your butt and saying you're not in the mood to do it today. Procrastination is the key to failure, so don't procrastinate. Get it done, and don't worry: I'm going to show you exactly how to get the results you most desire. In the next chapter, I'll explain how I learned to stop making excuses and start building my life around the Wellness Tripod.

CHAPTER 3

My Fitness Journey

I started my fitness journey about twenty-five years ago, as a chubby kid in the South Bronx. When I say "chubby," I mean I had freakin' man boobs and a gut. I got picked on plenty at school because of my weight. My aunt used to make fun of my breasts: "Donovan, I'm gonna get you a training bra for Christmas." She didn't mean any harm, and frankly I had the chest for it.

I was eight years old when my family moved to the Bronx from Jamaica. My father fixed cars, and my mother was a home attendant for senior citizens. They both worked very hard and were good at what they did, but money was always tight in our house. I wasn't a very needy kid, so I didn't put any pressure on my parents. I was always grateful for whatever I received.

Contrary to popular stereotypes of the inner city, my parents weren't crack addicts, criminals, or welfare recipients. They worked nonstop just to make ends meet. Though times were often tough, they always made certain that my sister and I never experienced hunger. There were days when I knew my folks were more stressed than others, but they never expressed that to us. Like all good parents, they made us believe everything was great.

Even though my mother worked two jobs all through my childhood, she still found time to exercise. As a kid I used to love watching her do her jumping jacks, sit-ups, and aerobic dancing in the living room.

My sister was three years younger than me, so I had to watch over her while my parents went to work. It felt great to take care of someone. I did everything I could as a big brother. Mind you, we argued and fought like two bulls in a pen. And yes, she tried to get me into trouble every time she got a chance!

At the neighborhood elementary school, my classmates made fun of my weight and my strong Jamaican accent. I got called "fat boy" and "black monkey." I was told to go back home to my country. I even got punched in the face one time, by a kid who just didn't like me. I went home feeling like crap. I quickly came to the realization that I needed to learn how to defend myself if I was going to survive this new world called America. So I asked my parents to put me in karate school, but they couldn't afford the fees at that time.

I soon realized that learning karate would not stop me from being bullied or teased. It was more about learning how to adapt and not allowing anyone to manipulate my mind or hurt my feelings. I was well adapted by the time I got to junior high school. I spent years developing the ability to tune out things that did not agree with my lifestyle. I kept only positive people around me who shared very similar likes and dislikes. I kept distant from those who were trouble.

One day my teacher asked me, "What is two plus one?" I told her, "Three," which I pronounced, "Tree." The entire class burst out laughing. One kid yelled out, "No, you fool, a *tree* is what grows outside. The answer is *three*!"

At first I didn't get why they were teasing me, because I couldn't see any difference between me and the other kids. I was small and they were small. I was black and they were black. I was in second grade and so were they. Finally my friend Lloyd explained that no one understood what the heck I was saying because of my accent. The funny thing is, they sounded just as strange to me as I did to them. I couldn't understand everything they were saying either. However, I did not make fun of them. Instead I chose to learn their version of the English language, full of words like "dope" and "fresh" that didn't mean what they meant back in Jamaica. It was like attending two schools at the same time.

DISCOVERING FITNESS

I went to church with my parents every Sunday. One day I looked around the congregation and realized that most of the folks around me were unhealthy. How was that possible? The pastor taught us that we needed to take care of our bodies because they were temples for our souls. We'd all say *amen*, but it seemed like no one was really following his words. Pretty much everyone in that church was fat and out of shape, including me, and nobody seemed to care.

For years I felt like I was living in a hamster wheel, with no way out. Everything changed when I turned thirteen, however. That's when my uncle Duncan came into my life and showed me what fitness was all about. My uncle looked like he just stepped out of a comic book. His body was and still is ripped to shreds, and he punched like Mike Tyson on steroids. He had a gym in his first-floor apartment on Anderson Avenue in the Bronx, downstairs from my parents' place. Nearly every day I would head down to Uncle Duncan's place and watch him work out with Keith, the building super.

At first I thought fitness training was only for adults. I just wanted to play Atari. That belief did not last long, however. Duncan took me under his wing and taught me the basics of weight lifting and self-defense. He helped me understand why people looked the way they did and what they could do to change their appearance. Duncan also taught me that true fitness requires mental and spiritual strength. With his help I learned not to let anyone or anything disturb my peace. I began talking to my friends about exercise and tried to explain how good it would make them look and feel. I wanted to help others feel the way I did.

The Bronx was a tough place to live in those days. It was the 1980s, and the inner-city crack epidemic was at its height. Every morning on my way to school I'd see empty green and blue vials littering the sidewalks. You'd see folks drunk at all times of the day. There were shoot-outs, too. One time I saw a man get stabbed by his wife. Grandmaster Melle Mel is an old friend and fellow warrior from the Bronx who helped invent hip-hop music through his groundbreaking work with Grandmaster Flash and the Furious Five. Melle Mel wrote memorably about that time in his 1982 track "The Message," where he describes the Bronx streets as a dangerous jungle. I was determined to survive and thrive in that jungle. And so I developed my No Excuses philosophy, based on my firm belief that true fitness depends on unyielding mental discipline as well as sound nutrition and regular exercise.

However, I found that most of my friends and family were lazy and uninterested in fitness. Though I still wanted to help people, I backed off on spreading the fitness gospel for a time. Instead I got into music. I played trombone and baritone sax in the marching band at Stevenson High School and even made it as a drum major. I connected with a whole new group of friends who were also music lovers. We started a rap group called the S.W.A.T. Team, short for Stacked with Annihilating Techniques. It was great for the time. I had a small music studio in my room and we would all get together to write lyrics and create original beats. We battled many other rappers and poets as well and took the trophy each and every time. It was fun while it lasted. Go, S.W.A.T. Team!

WORKOUTS AND HAIRCUTS

After I finished school, I supported myself as a barber and building contractor while I built up my business as a fitness coach. I learned carpentry, plumbing, and electrical work from an older gentleman named Glen Stewart. He was a Rasta from Trinidad, with a very small frame and a salt-and-pepper beard. Glen would buy homes in Brooklyn and the Bronx, fix them up, and resell them. He was hard, and he did not take any crap from me. I tried to argue with Glen one day and he shut me up immediately. "I did not choose to help you learn what I am teaching you. God did," he said. "Do not force me to go against his plans." After that I never talked back to Glen again.

My other trade was barbering. I dropped out of college to attend Atlas Barber School—I was already a barber in my community, but I wanted to learn how to cut all different types of hair, not just Afro texture. At nineteen I was earning $400 to $600 per week just from cutting hair. I set up a barbering station in a corner of my bedroom, and I drove my parents crazy with all the customers coming in and out of the house to get a haircut. My father complained the most, but he eventually became one of my clients. When I first started cutting hair, I gave him a horrific haircut. His co-workers at the garage made so much fun of him that he had to shave his head just to shut them up.

Barbering allowed me to help my parents financially. Eventually I became a full-time barber, making more money than my mother and father put together. I also began to combine fitness training and barbering. I used to hold push-up contests for customers to see who could do the most, with a discounted haircut for the winner. I spent hours talking about fitness and health to anyone who would listen. I started training people in the park for free, and I was so excited to see the results for both myself and them.

KICKBOXING WITH GREMENTHIA

My first paying client was a single mom named Grementhia Flournoy. The first time I visited her apartment in the Bronx, Grementhia opened the door, looked me straight in the eye, and gave me a big hug. Her apartment was strikingly clean and well organized. She seemed at peace in her surroundings. She moved easily and had no problem finding anything she needed. If you didn't know it already, you'd never guess that Grementhia was legally blind.

Squint as hard as you can, and then try to read the small print on a cereal box. That will give you an idea of what Grementhia sees every day. She can make out shapes and colors, but basically her world is one big blur. As I got to know Grementhia, I learned that she was dealing with a whole lot of challenges behind that serene façade. She had lost her sight about two years before we met and hadn't exercised since then. She was unemployed and raising a thirteen-year-old boy by herself. She weighed 237 pounds, suffered from depression and high blood pressure, and often had trouble sleeping because she was stressed out.

I started training Grementhia regularly, both at her home and in a nearby park. We did everything from strength training to kickboxing, which she especially enjoyed. Balance was a major challenge for Grementhia at first. Try standing on one leg with your eyes closed and then executing a roundhouse kick, and you'll have some idea of what kickboxing felt like for her. She also had trouble getting her head around the idea of intensity. As we trained she learned how to go faster and harder. Over time she mastered a full repertoire of kicks and punches, along with elbow and knee strikes.

It wasn't always smooth sailing. One day I came by Grementhia's house for training and noticed that her energy was way down. She seemed unhappy, but I didn't ask her what was wrong. I just said, "I can see you're not in the mood for a lot today, so when do you want to train next?" I didn't stress her; I didn't bother her; I just allowed the day to be the day.

I came to the house another day and found Grementhia looking exhausted. She told me that she hadn't slept at all the night before. "Tired or not, you're alive and breathing," I said. "Let's go!"

I had her do jumping jacks, sit-ups, push-ups, and squats, followed by our usual kickboxing routine. I burned her out, and I noticed she looked much better by the end of the session. Her adrenaline was pumping and her energy was up. By pushing herself through the workout, she had managed to ditch whatever was holding her down.

Grementhia still struggles with depression sometimes. But she keeps on pushing forward. Her weight has dropped to 180 pounds, and believe me when I tell you that she knows how to beat people's asses. Grementhia has developed into a seriously good kickboxer. She's fast, powerful, agile, and extremely flexible. She also has acute hearing, which helps compensate for her poor vision. When I throw a punch at her she can hear that movement and duck out of the way faster than a sighted person could.

When I'm going through tough times in my own life, I always think about Grementhia Flournoy. Her life proves that anyone can train their spirit, mind, and body to overcome major resistance. Grementhia may be blind, but she sees farther than most.

COMMITTING TO FITNESS

Along the way I met my beautiful wife, Ayana. She was a breath of fresh air from the moment I saw her walking on Baychester Avenue in the Bronx. Just like me, Ayana was a martial artist who loved to ride motorcycles. We sparred in the park on our first date, and until the children came we used to ride our bikes together all over the place.

Ayana and I got married and started a family. The bills started piling up, and though I was making money, I was not making enough. My barbering and contracting businesses both went downhill for a while, and Ayana had to pay the bills until I got back on my feet. I felt like a real loser, but I thanked God every day for blessing me with such a great woman.

Finally I decided to become a certified personal trainer. My first job was at an upscale gym in Manhattan. On my first day the other trainers warned me that I'd find it hard, even impossible, to sign up clients for private training. I've never really enjoyed being told that I can't do something, so I went out on the floor and chatted with a few members. By the end of that first day I had signed three new clients, which the other trainers and the gym manager thought was a miracle.

I learned a lot from working in that gym, but I didn't much care for its corporate atmosphere. I also didn't understand why personal training had to cost so much money, especially if the idea was to help people build better lives. I decided to move on and do my own independent thing in the Bronx. I handed out business cards advertising myself as the trainer who would come to you. Soon I was training at least twenty clients per week. I was grateful for all the business, but I still wanted to do more in the community. My clients could afford a personal trainer, but that wasn't true for most folks in the Bronx.

So I opened a community gym in a storefront on Prospect Avenue. My goal was to create a safe space for ordinary people to work out and learn about fitness. I fixed up the space myself, using the contracting skills Glen Stewart had taught me. I charged clients a $5 day rate to work out and trained several fitness coaches to help them. We organized fitness seminars led by celebrities like Dr. Oz, who had recently become my client, as well as New York Knicks basketball star John Starks and Broadway choreographer Stepp Stewart. We worked with local schools to organize training sessions for students. Soon the customers were pouring in like water.

Our slogan was "The Words 'I Can't' Do Not Exist." I constantly reminded my staff and clients that fitness starts in the mind and not the body. Clients would get frustrated because they weren't seeing results fast enough. "What's the hurry?" I would ask. They would reply that they needed to get fit before summer. When I asked why, they'd give me another answer, like "I want to look good in a bathing suit."

"How come?" I'd ask.

"So I can impress my boyfriend."

"Why do you want to do that?" And so on. When they had exhausted all possible responses, I would tell them that fitness has no deadline. Results come once you clear your thoughts and allow your body to simply be.

MY BROTHER DIAMOND

That kind of serenity doesn't grow by itself. It requires sustained mental and emotional discipline. I learned that lesson from a man named Diamond. He'd spent fifteen years in prison, getting out in his early thirties. He worked as a security guard and moonlighted as an exotic dancer, all the while building up his body at local gyms. The first time I saw him was on a subway train rolling underneath the Bronx. I was straphanging, and I saw this big guy sitting down who looked like the black Incredible Hulk. He was with a young woman. At a stop, an older white guy walked into the car and sat down opposite the Hulk. He had a bushy white beard that made him look like Santa Claus.

Santa said something to the Hulk—I'm not sure what it was, but the Hulk obviously felt disrespected. His voice got deeper and deeper, and he started growling all types of threatening things. Santa was just looking away, trying to defuse the situation, I guess.

Finally the Hulk stood up, and the whole car went quiet. He started walking back and forth with a tight fist, breathing heavily. Then he punched an extra-thick fortified pane of door glass, which shattered. The train pulled in to a stop, the doors opened, and the Hulk walked out. I saw his arm muscles pulsating like a heartbeat as he strode down the platform.

The next time I saw the Hulk, he was upset about his haircut. In those days my older brother Marvin and I used to run a little barbershop on Westchester Avenue, right around the corner from my new gym. In the basement below the shop I rigged up a martial arts studio where I practiced karate and jiujitsu. One day I was downstairs working out when I heard a commotion upstairs. One of my friends came running downstairs and said, "Yo, Donovan, there's a dude upstairs wants to beat up the barber!"

I ran up the stairs and saw the angry guy from the subway train yelling at one of my barbers, a young man named Drey. "What's going on?" I asked politely.

The Hulk whirled around and glared at me. "Who you, anyway?"

I explained that I was one of the owners, and I asked him again why he was upset. Apparently the barber had trimmed his hair too short, and he didn't want to pay for the cut. I told him I'd be more than happy to pay for his cut. "It's just hair," I added. "It'll grow back in a few days."

That just seemed to make him madder. He started asking all the other barbers and customers for a phone. Finally he grabbed a cell phone from a scared teenager and dialed a number.

"It's Diamond," he said. "Bring the hammer on down to that barbershop on Westchester."

Now, I knew Diamond wasn't talking about no hammer from Home Depot. He wanted his gun, and that meant I had to get serious with him. I told him to step outside, because we were going to take it to the next level.

So Diamond and I faced off on the sidewalk outside Marvin's Barber Shop. He was expecting to fight. I was ready to beat him down, but I always like to explore all possible alternatives to violence. So I explained that it was unacceptable for him to threaten deadly violence in my barbershop, a place that my wife and children visited every day. He quickly toned down. I told him to get back on the phone and squash that plan about the gun. He did that too.

Then I told Diamond that I was getting ready to open a new gym around the corner. "You've got an awesome physique," I said. "You might enjoy working out there." I told him to take a walk with me. I could see he was hesitant, but he followed me to the space I was building out in a former martial arts dojo on Prospect Avenue. I popped the lock and showed him all the new weights and machines that I was installing. All the while, I watched his energy go from tense to more relaxed.

A week later Diamond walked into the gym, paid his $5 at the front desk, and pumped some iron. On his way out the door he looked at me and said, "Yo, I'll be back." This was the guy who'd wanted to shoot up my barbershop a week before. Now he was working out in my gym!

Diamond became a regular after that. The next issue we had was over his habit of leaving his weights unracked after he was done using them. I told him to rack his weights so they'd be ready for the next user. I wanted to see if he was capable of following rules, or if he was going to get mad in the gym and act up again. He respected what I told him and started racking the weights.

A few weeks later I asked Diamond if he'd ever thought about becoming a personal trainer. I could tell he was interested, but he lacked confidence in himself. He said he didn't know anything about training people. "I'm here to teach you," I said. "I think you can be awesome." So he started training and found that he liked seeing folks groan and moan and helping them get stronger.

I gave him some fitness books to read. That's when I started seeing a whole new side of Diamond. He had a real love for studying and learning. He bought himself a notebook and started writing down all the different muscles and parts of the body. Pretty soon he was talking like he'd swallowed the dictionary.

One day Diamond and I were alternating on the bench press. He told me that nobody he'd worked with in gyms had ever pushed him the way I did, physically or mentally, and how much he appreciated having me in his life.

"I love you, man," he said. Then Diamond racked his weights, started crying, and gave me a big hug.

This was a guy who used to be ruled by his emotions, which was what got him into so much trouble. He learned how to stop and breathe. He learned how to think before he acted. That's one of the most important lessons that you'll learn in the No Excuses program.

CHAPTER 4

Mind

Fitness starts in the mind. Have you ever had one of those days when you wake up and feel like the world is mad at you for no reason? When you go through the day feeling like crap, and you do not understand why you feel this way? If your answer is yes, then you

> "A man is but the product of his thoughts. What he thinks, he becomes."
> —Mahatma Gandhi

need to realize that the world is still turning and it is paying you absolutely no attention. You are the one who chooses to feel like crap, and only you can choose to feel better.

We humans have a natural tendency to blame the world for all our problems and issues. It's almost never our fault. The truth is that while we all share responsibility for the world's troubles, you are solely responsible for your personal problems. You are the one who decides whether to eat breakfast or not, to turn left or right, to say yes or no.

We spend too much time blaming the present on the past, which in turn darkens our future. Remember, your mind can win or lose a battle. If you think negatively you can expect negative outcomes. So turn your mind around, think positive thoughts, and watch how good things start to happen.

As we've discussed, there's much more to fitness than dieting and working out. In order to maintain a healthy, sustainable lifestyle, you need resilience, emotional balance, and spiritual serenity. These are the building blocks of mental fitness.

DON'T FEAR PAIN

If I told you to go outside and run 10 miles right now, you might think I was crazy. But you already defeated yourself by thinking it was impossible. You have to tell yourself you can do anything. There is nothing you can't do. I personally love to take challenges that push me to the limit. It forces me to go beyond the threshold and embrace the pain.

There are many reasons why people fail at their exercise programs, but fear of pain is number one in my book. You can't be afraid of feeling pain during your workout. You must accept the pain and allow yourself to be present at all times. I always say, give me more! Your body can always find the energy to do one extra rep. Your mind will find the energy to just keep going. You must not get discouraged when you fail. Just tell yourself that you'll do better next time.

Yoga can help you let go and embrace the pain, allowing you to be present and go the extra mile. Some yoga poses require considerable physical strength, but mostly what's needed is mental strength. You have to hold each pose for a certain period, during which your only job is to clear your mind and breathe.

Once you begin to tell yourself that the pose hurts, you will immediately collapse. And yet the goal is not to push yourself to the point of injury. It's really about learning how to take control and push past the point where there is no more pain. Yoga mastery demonstrates the power of the mind. So does holding your breath underwater, or standing still like a statue for long periods. Before you can even attempt these things, you must train your mind to be strong and resilient.

HOW TO BUILD RESILIENCE

No matter what you do in life, success requires not just hard work but also the ability to take adversity in stride. All top athletes have the ability to come roaring back after any setback. The same is true for successful people in other occupations.

Here's the good news: Resilience is like a muscle, which means that you can strengthen it through exercise. There are innumerable ways to build muscular strength: lifting weights, swimming, riding a bicycle, practicing yoga, toting a backpack full of rocks. You should never wait for bad news from your doctor to start living a more healthy life. The same rules apply to building mental resilience.

Here are seven ways to build resilience:

1. **Learn from your mistakes.** Everybody screws up: It's part of being human. The key is to view every mistake as an opportunity to improve.
2. **Face reality.** Never turn your back on difficult problems and hope they will just go away. Trust me—they won't. Instead, confront your problems and solve them

one step at a time. Look at it this way: Every challenge is another doorway you must pass through on the way to success.

3. **Look ahead.** Instead of dwelling on bad things that happened in the past, concentrate on how your actions today will affect your future.

4. **Set reasonable goals.** Many of us tend to set unrealistic goals, which is a recipe for failure. If you've been sedentary your whole life, don't tell yourself that you're going to run a marathon next Saturday. Instead, set achievable goals. After you hit each milestone, set a new one. Get up right now and walk around the block a couple of times. Tomorrow, walk around the block a few more times. Once you have walking down, start jogging a little farther and for a little longer every day. Once you can jog for 30 minutes without too much strain, go out and run a 5K race, and then a 10K. Before you know it, that marathon will be in your sights!

5. **Look on the bright side.** Whenever I'm going through a tough time in my life, I always remind myself that people all over the planet are dealing with much more serious problems than mine.

6. **Lean on your friends.** I love talking to my very close friends whenever I get hit with a blow in my life. My friends tell me what I need to hear, not what I want to hear.

7. **Do what you say and mean what you do.** This one is pretty simple: Always follow through on your commitments, and never act halfheartedly. That applies to your work, your family, your friends, and your fitness program.

> Emotion: n. Disturbance of mind; mental sensation or state; instinctive feeling as opposed to reason.
> —Concise Oxford Dictionary

MENTAL FITNESS 101

If you can think it, you can and will achieve it.
If you aim at nothing, you will hit nothing.
Your outcomes are determined by your actions.

EMOTIONAL FITNESS

Now that you have started the process of building mental resilience, we can move on to the emotional side. We all have unique DNA, which means that no two people are exactly alike. What makes one person cry will make another laugh. What makes one person happy will make another angry. Even genetically identical twins are different in many ways, including fingerprints, birthmarks, hair patterns, and, most important, personalities.

Though humans are genetically different, we are all emotional creatures by nature. We all have emotions and we all use them one way or another. We communicate our thoughts emotionally, by crying, by laughing, and even through silence. Emotions are more powerful than a werewolf during a full moon. They can foster great outcomes. They can also cause absolute destruction among family and friends.

I'm not a psychotherapist, so I won't delve too deeply into the field of emotions. If you suffer from extreme depression, for example, then you should seek appropriate professional help. In this chapter, however, I do want to provide a set of simple, useful practices that will help boost your emotional fitness in a way that will buttress your No Excuses program.

When life gets tough, many of us let our emotions take over. It's not always the bad things that make us emotionally unstable. Positive events can have the same effect. For some, anxiety about a specific task such as finishing a term paper can cause more emotional damage than losing a job.

Emotional instability can cause undesirable or fatal behavior, such as abusing drugs and alcohol, eating an unhealthy diet, neglecting to exercise, hurting others, even suicide. Obviously, emotional instability tends to limit your ability to be strong and healthy. How can you hope to balance anything else in your life if you are emotionally off-balance?

Emotionally stable individuals handle hard knocks gracefully. They learn to accept situations for what they are, and they don't get overly stressed during difficult times. They tend to show resilience in everything they do. You can start to boost your emotional fitness right now by:

- **Surrounding yourself with positivity.** Find music you love, books that inspire you, people who make you happy all the time. This will allow you to think more clearly, with less room for gloomy thoughts.
- **Connecting with others.** Start by joining a discussion group on a topic that piques your interest. You can learn a lot about yourself by listening to someone else's experiences or even sharing your own experiences with a sympathetic audience.
- **Developing better eating habits.** This will help to reduce your level of guilt and keep you feeling healthier and more energized.

- **Avoiding drugs and alcohol.** I don't drink or take drugs, and that works for me. I'm not saying you can never have a glass of wine, but I strongly urge you to avoid abusing alcohol, which will damage every aspect of your health. The same is true for any recreational stimulant. Bottom line: Don't use chemicals to get high! Instead, learn to channel the exhilaration that comes from maintaining a healthy, positive lifestyle.
- **Exercising regularly.** Twenty minutes of high-intensity training a day for a maximum of 6 days per week can help you to reduce an enormous amount of stress, not to mention some excess body fat. The better you look, the better you feel, and vice versa.
- **Avoiding unnecessary expenses.** Try to live within your means and not beyond them.

STAY ON TRACK

Boosting your emotional health will also build your ability to stay motivated and committed to this program. How many times have you told yourself you were going to save more money, lose weight, or get a better job, only to give up?

The initial thought seems feasible and realistic. Your entire life is now dedicated to reaching that goal, and success seems right at your fingertips. Everything is at full throttle; not even Superman could slow you down. You buy books, read magazines, watch videos, and attend seminars because you're hungry for information that will help ensure your success. The more you learn, the hungrier you become. This is what it takes to succeed, and you are doing it.

And then you hit a wall. Your motivation flags, and you start reverting to the bad habits that made you want to change in the first place. Life starts to feel normal again. But is this the life you really want? There has to be an end point for bad habits, and that end point should be right now.

Failure is much easier than success. Most people want to be followers, not leaders. After all, followers don't face the consequences of failure in the same way that leaders do. It's so much easier to put the blame on someone else. This alone should explain why most of humanity is controlled by a tiny minority. There are many who come close to reaching their goals, and then they quit. That makes absolutely no sense to me. How about you?

Ask yourself this question: Do I want to succeed or do I want to be a failure? We all make mistakes, but you can't fall off track and never get back on just because you made an error. You started off strong, with nothing but the will to win. Each time you lose focus, you must fight to get that feeling back. The minute you give up is the minute you fail.

There is no room for failure in my life, and I won't accept failure from you. You are perfect only at making mistakes. But after every mistake you must get right back up, brush yourself off, and start again.

Here's a question I often ask my clients: I understand that failure often stops us from moving forward. And yet, don't you fail if you don't move forward? What would you do if failure wasn't an option? Would you open a business, go back to school, start a family, invest your money, go back to church, stop using harmful substances, and go to the gym?

Here's the bottom line: You must believe in whatever you attempt, be it getting a new job, asking somebody out on a date, or getting fit. Those who truly believe in their mission will always succeed. Without belief, there will be no success; you will only set yourself up for failure. I have personally tried to get involved in things that I did not believe in. For example, I once spent some time selling Amway products. Let's just say it didn't work out very well. It was easy to back out of that gig because I had no true belief in it. Without belief, there was no commitment.

Once you believe in yourself, you will find it much easier to deal with everyday challenges. So what if your body is sore? So what if your neighbor has a bigger house? So what if you lost your job or your spouse no longer loves you? It doesn't mean your life is over. You are the ruler of your life and you can get anything you desire. All you have to do is change your mind-set. That's how I became who I am today, and I'm not done yet. I'm still on a journey to total fitness that started twenty years ago with one very simple realization: There's no other way out of this pit except up.

SPIRITUAL FITNESS

Fitness begins and ends with a strong, healthy spirit. For me, spiritual fitness is not about following any particular religion or spiritual practice. Rather, it means understanding your place in the universe. It's about seeing how all things are connected, and how you are connected to all things.

A spiritually fit individual has a sense of peace, understands his or her purpose in life, and feels

"Your duty is to be, and not to be this or that."
—Ramana Maharshi

connected to others. In order to achieve spiritual fitness, you must first understand how the universe differs from you. Unlike you, the universe is designed to simply be. It does not create or destroy. It does not depend on anything in order to exist. It is always present, even when you are not. It does not rest, eat, drink, judge, or make errors.

The universe is not a place, person, or thing. It does not take sides in time of war. There are no cell phone numbers or e-mail addresses to reach the universe. It exists in you and you in it. Every time you let go of your feelings, whether good or bad, you simply let them go to the universe. It's that simple: Just give them to the universe.

Unfortunately you are not perfect and balanced like the universe. You sleep, eat, drink, judge, and make errors. You probably have a phone number and e-mail address where you can always be reached. You are known as the almighty human being. You are a king to many species, and lunch to a few.

Because nobody is perfect like the universe, we all need to work on building spiritual fitness. In essence, this means learning how to answer a simple question: Why do I live? Many of us live to please others. We pray to gods we don't believe in, say things we don't mean, drive cars we can't afford, and eat foods that we don't really like, all just to blend in with society. Some people are so skilled at dissimulation that they start believing their false lives are real. In short, they forget who they really are.

What is the point of existing if you can't be yourself? You commit spiritual suicide every time you kill the real you to satisfy the ego of others. So it's time to take a long look in the mirror, and I don't mean to check your makeup or hairline. Examine the real you. Open your eyes and tell yourself the truth about yourself.

Spiritual fitness is not measured in wealth, status, or possessions. Your house, job, or car can become your chain if you give it too much importance. And while I believe spiritual fitness is essential to overall health, you can't build it just by dieting and working out.

In order to build a strong, serene spirit, you must realize that you are the captain of your ship. Other than the Almighty, no force in the universe can make you or break you. No physical power can overcome the strength of your spirit. Don't let anyone use you as a vessel to dump negative energy or poisonous rubbish. You are not a garbage container. Avoid gossip, rumors, misleading accusations, and any other toxins that people might try to dump into your eardrums.

You must also refrain from pouring negative energy into other people. The person sitting in front of you is a perfect reflection of you, so be kind to yourself. Do not reject people who look or speak differently than you. Embrace them instead.

However, you shouldn't embrace someone just because of a smile, or because they make your heart feel good. There are many people out there who will pretend to be your friends. They will smile, call you nicknames, give you gifts, and even say they love you. They make you feel special and you love it. Is that what you really want, to feel special? You are obliged to make yourself feel special.

Don't depend on the actions of someone who is in your life only for the moment. Remember, your spirit is your true guide. Your heart can easily be broken by a phone call or the snap of a finger. By contrast, a strong spirit can mend a broken heart.

You can build spiritual fitness by:

- **Conscious breathing.** Breathing is a form of meditation because every breath affirms your connection to the universe. For a few minutes every day, focus only on inhaling and then exhaling. As you do, your mind will become quiet and serene.
- **Cultivating equanimity.** Know that every bad event will bring some good and vice versa. Keep reminding yourself that everything happens for a reason.
- **Accepting the inevitable.** You are not God, so you are not all-powerful. This means that you can't control every aspect of your life. Once you accept this reality, your mind will be more at ease and you will have more insight into the things you can change, such as your attitude, your nutrition, and your physical fitness.
- **Taking time for yourself.** Try to spend at least an hour per day on your own with no external disturbances such as radio, telephone, computer, or car. I know that's not always easy, but the spiritual payoff is immense. Meditation is a great way to take time for yourself. So is working out, gardening, going for a run, or walking in the woods with your dog.
- **Living for the moment.** You must enjoy every moment in your life and accept it as it comes. Look at your life as a blessing and not a curse. People often ask me why I'm always smiling. My answer: Because I'm alive and enjoying this very moment. I smile because I'm breathing, which is always preferable to the alternative.

Why do you live? I can't answer that question for you, but I will say that your spiritual purpose is like a puzzle. Once you connect the first few pieces, everything will fall into place. Here is an ancient hint to get you started on this quest: "To every thing there is a season, and a time to every purpose under the heaven" (Ecclesiastes 3:1). There is a time to sing, a time to cry, even a time to die. This moment is your time to live.

As your spiritual fitness grows, you will learn to be calm like the summer breeze. Your mind will flow like water. You will see more of the world for what it really is. Nothing will look pretty or ugly. It will just be present, right here, right now. In the process you will become healthier, less stressed, and filled with enough energy to light an entire city. So put your fears aside, silence those dark thoughts, and trust your spirit to guide you through your journey. Once your spirit is strong, everything else will follow.

TAKE A BREATH

Stop whatever you're doing, fill your lungs with air, and allow your abdomen to expand. Now exhale slowly and let your abdomen deflate back to its normal size. Feel your heart beat and your lungs move as the air passes through to keep your heart beating. You should feel revitalized just from that simple exercise. I did it as I wrote this section of the book, and I felt great.

CHAPTER 5

Food

You need to pack your parachute properly before you jump out of a plane. Similarly, you can't feel and look good if you don't eat a healthy, balanced diet. You may not be gearing up to win the Ultimate Fighting Championship or go full throttle in the next world war, but this is still war—the war on obesity. It's time for you to start winning the battle that so many Americans lose on a daily basis.

> "The doctor of the future will give no medicine, but will instruct his patient in the care of the human frame, in diet and in the cause and prevention of disease."
> —Thomas Edison

Food is a quiet addiction. As a kid in the South Bronx back in the 1980s, I learned to recognize the zombielike affect of a hard-core crack addict. Food addiction, on the other hand, has no direct symptoms. Just because someone looks fit doesn't mean they eat right. Of course, the same thing applies to those who are overweight; it does not mean they eat wrong. Many of us eat because we can and not because we have to. We eat during any form of celebration, when we are stressed, even when we are tired.

And yet food is not the enemy; you are. It's all up to you to make the change. I learned how to control my nutritional intake and I will share my journey with you. You will learn how to control your attitude toward food and how to say *no*!

Temptation is everywhere. The industrial food complex bombards us with images of delicious food 24/7. I myself find it hard to say no sometimes, just because it all looks and tastes so darn good. The brain tends to interpret visual stimuli as a prompt to take action. We begin to lose control and start drooling like hungry lions. We forget all about our mission to stay healthy and eat clean.

After satisfying that craving comes the guilt. Many people try to deal with the guilt by telling themselves they will just do an extra hour in the gym. That hardly ever happens, but it sounds good to your brain at the time. Another way we lose control is simply by making up a ton of reasons why we can't go to the gym. There's always the next day, right? It always sounds so much better when we say we'll go tomorrow. *Boom!* Tomorrow is here and you still didn't go to the gym. You keep on telling yourself you will make it up. All of a sudden 2 months have passed, you're 10 pounds overweight, and you *still* haven't made it to the gym. (Yikes!)

In some ways we humans are simple creatures. When we see something that appeals to us, we do whatever it takes to get it. Even if it's bad for our health, we tend to go for it anyway. Trust me, I have never seen anyone go crazy for a piece of squash or say, *Hey, let's celebrate and get some kale with spinach!* Chances are that the object of your craving will be bad for your health. There are those who crave veggies, but like the golden tabby tiger, they are very rare.

In this chapter you'll learn how to buy and prepare healthy food without busting your budget or turning your kitchen into a disaster zone. This is not about starving yourself or following the latest diet fad. Rather, it's about eating a balanced, sustainable diet that includes protein, fat, carbohydrates, fiber, vitamins, and minerals.

I'll show you how to prepare healthy, portable meals in advance, so that you (and your wallet) are not at the mercy of the industrial fast-food complex when you're out and about. I'll also provide shopping lists, instructions on navigating an American supermarket (**note:** avoid the middle aisles, where most of the junk food is found), and healthy, delicious, easy-to-prepare recipes inspired by the savory Caribbean cuisine that I ate growing up in Jamaica and the South Bronx.

Every day you should eat six light meals or meal replacements, such as my special Funky Kingston Smoothie (recipe on page 158), so that your metabolism is always working at its optimal fat-burning level. Your metabolism is the sum of all the physical and chemical processes by which energy is made available to your cells. The key is to feed your body about every 2 hours. At this pace your body metabolizes food efficiently, extracting the energy that it needs and discarding waste. If you allow much more than 2 hours to elapse between meals, your body will go into starvation mode and start storing fat.

Here is a question I always ask when I speak at health seminars. Why do you spend hundreds if not thousands of dollars feeding your car? You buy the best gas, oil, paint, air freshener, tires, and so on. Is it because your car has a certain market value and you want to keep that value up? If that's the case, then how much do you think you are worth? I am willing to bet that you would never fill your car's gas tank with sand. If you did, you'd be considered a real idiot. So why would you put junk into your body?

Living healthy means taking the time to care for yourself, with no excuses. I am convinced that nutrition is the secret to staying fit and that its neglect is the cause of disease. You can't transform your body without focusing on nutrition.

PROGRESS, NOT PERFECTION

The No Excuses program is not about 100 percent compliance. Rather, it's about heading in the right direction. I always say that as far as food goes, my life is 80 percent clean. This means I leave enough room to enjoy my favorite junk foods without compromising my general mission.

I used to eat a lot of red meat because I thought I needed it to build up my muscles. Fifteen years ago I stopped eating red meat, just because it felt like the right thing for me. Don't worry, I'm not going to try to convince you to stop eating meat or to eliminate all sugary and fattening foods. Instead I'll provide healthy, delicious alternatives to the stuff that's bad for you. And guess what? The more you eat healthy, the more you'll want to eat healthy. You won't have to deprive yourself.

You can start by finding healthy substitutes for less-than-healthy foods that you crave. You love milk shakes? My Protein Power Hit (recipe on page 159) is a tasty, healthy alternative to shakes that are full of sugar and fat. Instead of pancakes slathered with industrial syrup, try my PB Wafflewich on page 168. Instead of inhaling that big bucket of ice cream, try a scoop of sherbet with mixed fruits. If that's not appealing, add some fruit or granola to a single scoop of ice cream.

Let's say you like to drink soda three or four times a day. Don't make the mistake of telling yourself that you are going to just stop drinking soda forever. Instead, cut those four sodas down to two. Replace the other two with freshly squeezed orange juice or a fruit smoothie. Alternatively, you can cut back to two sodas but increase their volume by using the half and half method. It's simple: just pour half of each soda into a cup and replace the other half with water. The key is to avoid all-or-nothing propositions. Transformation is about making choices, and I will give you options to make the right ones for you. Think of your diet as a continuum ranging from unhealthy to healthy. You want to keep sliding toward the healthy end of the spectrum. Progress, not perfection, is key.

MYTHBUSTER

Myth: I don't need to exercise, because my diet will keep me skinny.
Fact: An exercise regime is essential to maintain weight loss. Also, dieting doesn't produce the same long-term health benefits as exercise.

FORGET WILLPOWER

Although most folks know what's good or bad for them, many of us find it very hard to do the right thing when it comes to nutrition. So how do you develop willpower? I must tell you the truth and nothing but the truth. I don't believe in willpower at all. Willpower is merely a shorthand way of saying *I am going to eat this junk later, and I am going to eat a lot of it.* Much like dieting, willpower is just a temporary fix.

When it comes to nutrition, you should focus less on willpower and more on lifestyle change. Here's a great example. The New Year comes around once a year, and every year thousands resolve to stop drinking, eating cake, or smoking cigarettes. We are all familiar with these so-called resolutions.

You apply willpower for 3 weeks or even 3 months straight. You're doing great. Every time you feel the urge to eat that cake or smoke that cigarette, willpower kicks in and you refrain. Then you get invited to a birthday party. You arrive at the party and see a huge cake made with vanilla and chocolate fudge, drizzled with chocolate chips, topped with strawberries, soaked in syrup. It has your name written all over it. Your mouth begins to salivate, but wait! Through a massive effort of will, you remain in control.

As the night wears on, you watch the other guests laughing and eating that cake. Every few minutes the question from hell arises: "Do you want some of this cake?" Followed by: "It's so good!" Your resolve weakens by the minute. At last comes the breaking point. You can't take this anymore. Just this one time, it won't hurt you at all. You'll resume that no-cake regime—wait for it—tomorrow!

Here's some advice. Instead of depending on willpower to keep you out of trouble, avoid situations where you have to fight temptation. It's like fighting an army by yourself. No matter how hard you fight, you'll eventually lose the battle. Sooner or later you will get tired and give up. Willpower is just a temporary fix. If your goal is long-term health and fitness, you must reboot your lifestyle. You have to want this badly enough to change a whole range of habits, including the food you eat, the society you frequent, the music you listen to, even the clothes you wear.

Do you have friends who encourage you to gorge on fast food like they do? Stop hanging out with them, at least at mealtimes. Do you associate particular songs with late-night food binges? Delete them from your playlist. Do you wear baggy clothes to hide those rolls of fat? Try more form-fitting outfits. You'll be amazed how exhibiting your physical imperfections will motivate you to eat properly.

If you want to be healthy, you must eat healthy. I can't stress this enough: Nutrition is 80 percent of your results. You should do your best to avoid processed sugars (including artificial sweeteners), salty foods, saturated fats, high-fructose corn syrup, and alcohol. Instead, include more water, vegetables, fruits, whole grains, vitamins, legumes, and lean meats in your diet. Once you do, your energy level will skyrocket and your brain will function at peak performance.

HOW I LEARNED TO EAT

Remember I told you that I used to be chubby as a kid? Growing up in a Jamaican household in the Bronx, I ate oxtails, curry goat, tripe, cow liver, kidney, fried fish, rice, and a whole lot of flour. My mother's cooking tasted so good that it was impossible to believe it could be bad for me. Plus, I didn't have a lot of dietary choices in those days. I could either eat what Mom put on the table, or go hungry.

Then I grew up, left home, and became a personal trainer. But I still struggled with my diet. I'd get sudden cravings for M&M'S, nachos, carrot cake with icing, Snickers bars, McDonald's, fried chicken, and Chinese food laced with flavor-enhancing mono-sodium glutamate. I was a personal trainer who ate like an idiot. I wish I could go back in time and punch myself in the head.

I also worked out a lot, so I didn't put on weight. But my poor diet was stopping my body from reaching its full potential. Of course I noticed differences in my shape, but the way I looked didn't reflect the number of hours I spent training every week. Though I grew stronger and gained muscle mass, my abdominal muscles were still not defined enough and my mirror muscles (chest, arms, shoulders, back) weren't popping the way I wanted them to.

I eventually came to that disgusting place known as a plateau. Although I continued to work out, I stopped progressing. I fed my internal organs nothing but fatty foods, which is a great way to die young. Folks would ask, "Why are you eating that? Aren't you a personal trainer? Is that good for you?" My response was always: "I'm fine, and I train more than five days per week so I'll burn it off in no time." They would look at me in amazement and say, *"Okay!"* I must have sounded like a real clown.

I began to look in the mirror, and I was not happy with what I saw. That was my guilty conscience kicking in. I stopped enjoying my workouts because I knew that my eating habits were sabotaging my results. I wasn't getting enough rest or drinking enough water. I was bored to death and had no motivation at all. People began to notice my unhappiness. My mind was going around in circles and my body no longer emitted the essence of a fit individual.

I started to study nutrition and found many different points of view. One expert would tell me to eat this and the next expert would tell me not to. The more I learned the hungrier I became for more information. Finally I discovered integrative nutrition, which doesn't push any specific diet or style of eating. Rather, integrative nutrition is a holistic approach to eating that focuses on balance and portion control. It teaches that healthy nutrition is all about being sensible and controlled. Basically it's the old Greek ideal: everything in moderation.

I am proud to tell you that I managed to shed my crazy lifestyle and come to my proper senses. Now I eat clean most of the time, which means that I avoid processed foods. Our bodies were not designed to consume the chemicals that processed-food manufacturers add to extend shelf life, boost flavor, and widen profit margins. Instead I eat mainly natural, minimally processed foods: fruits, vegetables, legumes, brown rice, and fish. I still leave some room for junk food, because I like my treats every now and then. And I've found that my clients progress much faster when they eat healthy. Common results include lower blood pressure and cholesterol, no asthma, and a tremendous loss of excess body fat. All this can be yours if you combine regular exercise with sound nutrition.

Integrative nutrition is not about starving yourself or following the latest fad diet. Whether you're a vegan, a meat eater, or something in between, make sure to choose fresh, natural foods that supply a balance of protein, complex carbohydrates, fiber, vitamins, and healthy (unsaturated) fats. Avoid refined sugars and alcohol, and eat plenty of fresh fruits and vegetables. For more specific food-shopping tips, see the pantry list on page 189.

Above all, don't overeat. According to legend, the philosopher Aristotle taught his young student Alexander that he should always get up from the table feeling that he could still eat a little more. That boy went on to conquer the entire known world, and today we call him Alexander the Great. Surely Alexander's diet had something to do with his success.

THE CURSE OF ABUNDANCE

Our Stone Age ancestors had very limited food supplies. They didn't have 24-hour supermarkets or fast-food joints. They couldn't open the freezer to get a bowl of ice cream. They hunted their meat and grew their fruits and vegetables, or else gathered them in the woods. Unlike modern food addicts, who live to eat, our ancestors ate to live. In order to survive the harsh winter season when food was scarce and hunting almost impossible, they stocked up on food during the summer and fall. Failure to plan ahead meant death from starvation.

Nowadays it's a whole different ball game. We have food by the ton. All we have to do is order from a website, and *boom*, our meals arrive at the door in a matter of hours. We indulge our gluttony by eating until we can't eat any more. Every year, roughly a billion tons of food get lost or wasted around the world, according to the UN Food and Agriculture Organization. Every year, consumers in rich countries like the United States throw away about 222 million tons of food, or nearly as much as the total annual food production of sub-Saharan Africa.

When was the last time you heard a doctor recommend the American diet? The standard acronym for the food that most Americans eat is SAD (Standard American Diet). It includes enormous quantities of refined flour, sugar, and processed foods. Think about that for a second before you read any further. SAD: That is not good at all.

So how can you build healthier eating habits? For most of us, it's easier to pick up a slice of cake than a bowl of vegetables. But you can overcome this mind-set just like I did. You just need to want it so bad that you will do almost anything to get there, including opting out of that easier choice.

HOW MANY CALORIES?

Other than algebra, the most confusing topic I know is how many calories a person should consume on a daily basis in order to lose weight. I haven't found the perfect answer, but I will share some important information on calorie consumption that will help you make your own decision.

It takes 3,500 calories to equal 1 pound of fat. Each person's metabolism is different, but let's say you consume 2,000 calories a day, or 14,000 calories in a week (2,000 x 7 = 14,000). At that rate you can store up to 4 pounds of fat per week if you don't burn more calories than you consume. However, if you create a small calorie deficit by cutting 500 calories out of your daily diet, you can lose 1 pound of fat per week (500 x 7 = 3,500).

Everybody likes to talk about calories, but weight loss is really about balance. We hear a lot about empty calories versus healthy calories, but what's the real difference? A calorie is simply the measurement of energy generated from food. It's the energy needed to increase the temperature of 1 gram of water by 1 degree Celsius. Do you remember the trick question about which is heavier, a ton of bricks or a ton of feathers? What was your answer? I believe a calorie is a calorie just the same as a ton is a ton.

The problem with weight gain is not necessarily the types of foods we eat, but the number of calories we consume. Mind you, I'm not suggesting that you can live on bacon and ice cream as long you restrict your overall calorie intake. You might not gain weight on that diet, but you'll be on the fast track to diabetes and heart disease. I'm also totally opposed to extreme dieting, which deprives the body of vital nutrients. If you consume too few calories, you'll lose weight but not in the right way. You will shed water and muscle rather than fat. And any weight loss will likely be ephemeral.

It's far better to eat a healthy, balanced diet and to limit how much you eat in one serving. Your body can metabolize no more than 500 calories per meal. This means that your cells have the capacity to use no more than 500 calories from any one meal as energy. Any excess calories will typically get stored as fat, which is your body's way of putting away some energy for a rainy day. So if you ingest 700 calories in a single meal, you will probably store 200 of those calories as fat. That's why you should spread your calories out by eating five small meals throughout the day. You must also follow a work-out program that will challenge your body to achieve its full potential. The combination of a sound diet with proper exercise will boost your metabolism and allow it to burn those calories.

BUILDING A HEALTHY DIET

There is a fine line between healthy and unhealthy. You can go either way in no time;

it's just that one is a little easier to get to than the other. I'll say it again: You have to want it so bad that you will do almost anything to get there.

You may feel like you don't have time to make better food choices. Well, I say you do. If you found time to read this book, then you can definitely find time to eat properly. I know time is short and daily responsibilities claim much of your attention. Everything is one big wheel once your body comes out of that temporary sleep coma. Your day begins and ends, and then you have to repeat the whole thing all over again. You ask yourself, when will this madness end? When will I have time to get fit and healthy? Is it too late for me to make a change?

I have great news: It's not too late to get your body in tip-top shape. There is no reason why you can't lose those unwanted pounds or gain the extra muscle you've been craving for so long. Despite your busy schedule, you can still find the time to exercise and eat sensibly. I don't expect you to become a vegan or vegetarian. I just want you to make better food choices.

Develop a balanced program of diet and exercise that will optimize your body's fat-burning system. Avoid crash diets that deprive your body of vital nutrients. Leave drugs and weight-loss pills alone, and make sure to limit each meal to no more than 500 calories. Don't forget, it took time to put on the weight and it will take some time to lose it. Keep on moving and stop at no cost.

Here are ten steps to a healthier diet. I expect you to follow them to the letter. You won't need to count calories or know how much sugar each meal contains. All you have to do is read and follow the steps.

STEP 1: Eliminate all refined sugars from your diet

Take a moment to look through your refrigerator and pantry. Now throw out anything that contains refined sugar, which is toxic for several reasons: It converts to fat in the body, it destroys brain cells, and it increases your chances of becoming diabetic. Instead, use natural sweeteners like agave and honey. I know you almost closed the book and demanded a refund. *Did he just say no sugar? Is he crazy?* If you want it bad enough like I did, you will have to make the commitment.

Nearly all packaged foods contained refined sugars. However, food manufacturers use sugar in many different forms. Here's a cheat sheet:

Refined Sugars to Avoid

"OSE" SUGARS	"OL" SUGARS	OTHER SUGARS
dextrose	manitol	cane juice
fructose	sorbitol	cane sugar
galactose	xylitol	corn sweetener
lactose		corn syrup
levulose		dextrin
maltose		granulated sugar
saccharose		high-fructose corn syrup
sucrose		malt syrup
xylose		maltodextrin
		rice syrup

STEP 2: Make a list

Now that you've purged refined sugar from your kitchen, it's time to prepare a grocery list. Make sure to break your list down into sections that are easy to understand, such as meats, vegetables, fruits, dairy, grains, seasonings, beverages, and miscellaneous. With a list you'll find it easier to shop without overspending or buying the wrong foods.

Note: Organic food is certainly healthier than nonorganic food because it contains few or no harmful additives. But it can be pricey, so I'm not going to preach the organic gospel. If you can afford to go organic, great. I particularly recommend buying the organic versions of thin-skinned fruits such as apples and berries, because pesticides and other chemicals pass into them easily. The organic label matters less for thick-skinned fruits like bananas, oranges, and grapefruit, because the skin keeps out the chemicals (also, people tend not to eat banana peels). But if your budget doesn't stretch that far, don't worry about it. You can eat a very healthy diet without ever going near the organic food section.

STEP 3: Go shopping

The true test begins at your friendly local supermarket. Bring your list and make sure you buy enough food for the entire week. One word of advice: Never shop on an empty stomach. Instead, snack on a piece of fruit or a peanut butter sandwich on whole wheat bread with natural fruit spread. You will be fed and ready to take on the world after a nutritious snack.

Here's another great rule of shopping: In most supermarkets, you'll want to stay in the outside aisles. The middle aisles are where you find enemy foods like cookies, chips, and ice cream cake. Recently some of the supermarket chains have caught on to this secret, so they've started to place healthy products like oatmeal, honey, agave, and high-fiber cereals in the middle aisles, forcing you to run a gauntlet of terrible food in order to find the good stuff. But in general you'll still find healthier, less-processed food in the outside aisles. (See the pantry list on page 189.)

STEP 4: Prepare your meals ahead of time

If you were going camping deep in the woods, you'd pack enough food to ensure your survival, right? The same goes for everyday life. If you leave your house without pre-pared food, you'll be tempted to grab the fastest meal you can find, which will more than likely be unhealthy. This is how we all make fatal errors that sabotage our prog-ress. The solution? Prepare your foods ahead of time.

Don't cook for just 1 day. Instead, prepare enough food to last at least 5 days out of the week. Make sure each meal consists of protein, complex carbohydrates, and healthy fats, which are the key elements of a balanced diet. Use airtight containers to section off your weekly food supply. Label them accordingly so you can know what you are eating each day. Simply place them in the freezer, and *boom*! Your weekly food needs are cov-ered. Every morning, just open the freezer and take out your day's worth of food, which will normally include a midmorning snack, lunch, a midafternoon snack, and maybe dinner if you work really late. (I'm assuming you eat breakfast at home.)

Starting on page 157 you'll find some of my favorite recipes to get you started. You shouldn't need more than 1 hour to prepare meals for the entire week. An hour for a week's worth of food is not bad at all, plus you will save a ton of money. You'll also know exactly what goes into your meals, which is not the case when you eat at restaurants.

STEP 5: Buy a portable cooler

Okay, so now you have your food ready for the week. Now you need a portable cooler big enough to hold each day's meals and transport them safely. Coolers come in all shapes and sizes. You can go old school with a cooler that requires a pack of ice, or you can go all Star Trek with a model that plugs into your car's 12-volt outlet. Coolers also come in different colors and designs, so you can certainly use your cooler to make a fashion statement. You don't need to go to work or school with a Scooby-Doo lunch box, unless that happens to be your thing.

You will never need to stop at your local deli or fast-food spot again. All you have to do is open your cooler, reach, grab, and eat. Clean, fresh, and made by you. What else could you ask for, except maybe a million dollars in cash?

STEP 6: Prepare a schedule

Create a daily schedule that will prompt you to exercise and eat at the proper times. Input the information in your phone calendar and set it to auto-reminder. This will be your accountability alarm. You must also write down your workout schedule and post it someplace inescapable, like your bathroom mirror or the inside of your front door.

Now that you've set up a reminder system, the rest is up to you. It's very important to follow your schedule to the letter. Don't miss meals! Missing meals will push your body into starvation mode, which encourages it to store fat. If not fed on a consistent basis, your body will shut off the fat-burning furnace known as your metabolism, which converts the food you eat to energy.

STEP 7: Drink plenty of water

Water is the body's transport system and the key element in life. It keeps your blood flowing, nutrients moving, and waste leaving your body. Water is also the body's cooling system. It regulates body temperature by redistributing heat from active tissues to the skin and then cooling you off via perspiration. If you don't drink enough water, you'll become dehydrated and your brain will not function at its best. Thirst is an obvious sign of dehydration. Other symptoms include cracked lips and skin, headaches, constipation, dizziness, diarrhea, dry mouth, no tears when crying, and loss of consciousness. Needless to say, you can avoid all these symptoms by drinking plenty of water throughout the day.

Body types vary, so it's hard to say exactly how much water you should drink every day. A good rule of thumb is that you should slurp down half an ounce of water per pound of body weight if you're sedentary, or 1 ounce of water per pound if you're very active. Here's a quick formula:

Sedentary range: body weight (pounds) x 0.5 (ounce) = ounces of water per day
Active range: body weight (pounds) x 1 (ounce) = ounces of water per day
Example: Someone who weighs 150 pounds should drink between 75 and 150
    ounces of water per day, depending on her level of activity.

STEP 8: Consume 25 to 30 grams of fiber per day

I know folks don't like to talk about going to the bathroom, but it's a necessary part of life as well as a great health indicator. Fiber helps your body get rid of waste and keeps your colon clean and healthy. Undigested fiber stays inside the intestines, either whole or in gel form. This helps keep your colon track nice and clear, like the highways after rush hour.

Once you increase your fiber intake, your bowel movements will become easier, with little or no strain. To achieve this happy state, you should eat 25 to 30 grams of fiber every day. You can get fiber from fruits, vegetables, bran cereal, oatmeal, nuts, and brown rice, as well as nutritional supplements. Always check with your doctor before using any supplements. Food should always be your first choice, and supplements your second.

There are two different types of fiber: *Soluble fiber* attracts water and turns to gel during digestion. It's found mainly in fruits, oat bran, peas, lentils, and vegetables. Soluble fiber can help lower cholesterol, which in turn reduces your risk of heart disease. *Insoluble fiber* is found in foods such as whole grains and vegetables. It adds bulk to your stool, helping it to pass more quickly.

Note: Pay strict attention to the shape and color of your stool. It should have the shape of a banana. Normal, healthy stools should be brown in color, indicating proper levels of bile. Grayish stools indicate a possible block in the flow of bile. Black stools are normally caused by internal bleeding or excessive iron intake. (Consult your physician in either case.)

STEP 9: Take your vitamins

Vitamins are essential to life. They help us fight off disease by building a stronger immune system. They also help to increase red and white blood cell counts, which means more energy throughout the day. All living creatures depend on vitamins to stay strong and powerful.

Our ancestors didn't need vitamin supplements because their food contained all the necessary vitamins. In the age of industrial food production, that's sadly no longer true. As the world's population grows, demand for food increases. To keep up with this demand, food producers have increasingly been growing crops with chemical fertilizers and feeding growth hormones to livestock. As a result, many of the foods we eat are filled with chemicals and hormones to the point that they lack the enzymes needed to produce vitamins. Though we can get the majority of our vitamins from eating a healthy and balanced diet, it's still necessary to take supplementary vitamins.

I personally like the convenience of multivitamins, and I prefer liquid vitamins to pills because liquids reach my bloodstream faster. It's important to note, however, that there's no one-size-fits-all solution when it comes to vitamins. Your doctor can help you design a sound vitamin regime based on your age, gender, diet, and body type.

Here's a list of the most important vitamins and their basic functions:

- Vitamin A promotes vision and healthy bone growth.
- Vitamin B1 helps metabolize carbohydrates and increase energy.
- Vitamin B2 boosts red blood cell production, which increases energy.
- Vitamin B3 stimulates strong and healthy skin.
- Vitamin B5 helps to release energy from foods.
- Vitamin B6 metabolizes protein and improves nervous system performance.
- Vitamin B9 (folic acid) speeds the production of red blood cells.
- Vitamin B12 helps to break down fatty acids, which increases energy and inhibits fat storage.
- Vitamin C helps to strengthen connective tissue, bones, and teeth.
- Vitamin D helps to build strong teeth and bones.
- Vitamin E protects the body's cells and maintains healthy red blood cells.
- Vitamin K is essential to the blood-clotting process.

STEP 10: Get enough sleep

I know you are anxious to get your body in tip-top shape. And yet you're so busy that there seems to be little or no time in the day for exercise. The days all blend together, and your hours seem shorter by the second. If that's how you feel, then you're probably not getting enough sleep. This is where most people go terribly wrong. Though I mentioned that nutrition is 80 percent of your results, sleep is also vital. Your body must be well rested to function properly.

Lack of sleep will lower your body's resistance to disease and damage your fitness. Your energy level will always be low, discouraging you from going to the gym or preparing meals ahead of time. How can you do all that with no energy?

You must make sure to get anywhere between 6 and 8 hours of sleep daily. I sleep about 6 hours a night—anything more makes me feel over-rested. Figure out how much sleep you need, and get it! Exhaustion will eventually force your body to shut down and sleep on its own, but that's not a good thing. You must consciously allow your body to relax comfortably into its sleep stages. If you do, you'll feel rejuvenated and ready to take on the world.

BONUS STEP: Have a little fun!

To be successful you must ensure that this entire journey is fun. If you have to constantly fight an urge, you will eventually lose. So leave a little room to enjoy a cheat meal. (Notice I did not say a cheat *day*!) It could be a vegan chocolate chip cookie, veggie pizza, or one scoop of ice cream. The idea behind the cheat meal is to feed your urge so you can then comfortably resume your healthy routine.

If you can do without a cheat meal, then more power to you. However, if you cannot go without a cheat meal, then by all means enjoy it with a big smile, from ear to ear.

HOW TO MEASURE PROGRESS

The best way to gauge progress in a fitness program is by periodically measuring your waist, hips, thighs, arms, and chest. You should also track your body mass index (BMI). One note of caution: BMI is a good proxy for overall health, but it doesn't distinguish between fat and lean mass. That's why you should also monitor your body-fat percentage, using a body-fat analyzer, available for less than $100 at your local pharmacy or nutrition store. (Most gyms and personal trainers will also measure your body-fat percentage as part of their service.)

Another great way to judge your results is simply by keeping track of how your clothing fits your body. Find or purchase a pair of jeans that's at least two sizes smaller than you are. Try them on once a month and mark down how far they come up past your thighs or how close the buttons are to closing. Before you know it, you'll be wearing those jeans right out the door!

LOSE THAT SCALE

Let me get right to the point. I need you to smash your bathroom scale with a sledge-hammer and then throw it in the trash. A scale is like a bad friend who wants nothing but the worst for you. It will tell you one of two things: Either you didn't lose any weight or you didn't lose enough. If there is any satisfaction to be gained from climbing on a scale, it's usually short-lived.

Why is the scale so important to you? Why do you feel like you've achieved something when you see a lower number? A scale is not the best way to judge your results. You need to look past the scale and focus on your physical performance. You can do 50 jumping jacks now compared to only 10 a month ago. You could complete only 2 push-ups, and now you can do 10 push-ups. Your jeans fit better, and a flight of stairs is no longer your worst enemy.

Do you see where I'm headed here? A scale will only disappoint you and make you feel like you are wasting your time when you are actually doing great. It probably took you 5 seconds to read the last paragraph. In those 5 seconds, I'm willing to bet that at least a hundred Americans quit their fitness program because the scale said they gained weight or didn't lose the weight they wanted to lose. *The scale is the devil disguised as your friend.*

STOP MAKING MISTAKES

This is your year to finally break the fat cycle and stop making crazy-ass mistakes, like skipping workouts and washing down that jumbo bag of peanut M&M'S with four glasses of wine. Obviously, we're all human and we all make mistakes. If you learn to kick yourself in the butt every time you mess up, however, you will make fewer mistakes.

Every day is a new day, but that doesn't mean you should mess up on your nutrition today with the mind-set that you are going to do better tomorrow. That only creates bad habits. Once bad habits take over, it becomes far more difficult to maintain a healthy regime.

Clients often tell me that they feel bad because they ate wrong. I used to reply, "No problem; there's always tomorrow." What the hell was wrong with me? I should have said, "Why did you mess up, and what was going through your thick skull? You've messed up enough times in your life. It's time to step away from the cake and alcohol. Instead, pick up some weights or go for a walk or run."

Fitness mistakes are dangerous because your body is unforgiving when it comes to storing fat. As a matter of fact, it will hold on to as much fat as possible if you permit it. So it's up to you to force your body to become a fat-burning furnace.

That's really not difficult. You need to eat lots of fruits, vegetables, and lean meats, you need to drink plenty of water, and you need to train your butt off. Above all, stop telling yourself that you can't eat right and exercise because it sounds too hard or you don't have time to go to the gym. These are merely excuses, sent by Satan from the pit of hell to limit your success.

Lastly, you need to stop giving up on yourself. You have more push in you than you think. So look in the mirror and ask yourself these questions: *Who am I? Am I happy? What is my problem? How long do I want to live?* After that, take a deep breath and keep reading. I'm going to show you exactly what it takes to achieve all your fitness goals.

CHAPTER 6

Exercise

Whenever I pick up some weights, punch a heavy bag, or go bike riding, I feel a great sense of joy and completion. I feel amazing knowing that I did my exercise for the day, leaving me free to spend time with my kids, write, lead a cardio-sculpt class, or simply get some well-deserved rest. Exercise plays the role of my therapist when I'm down and my motivator when I'm trying to run a 7-minute mile.

Some of my clients feel the same way I do about exercise. They train with me 3 days out of the week and do another 3 days on their own. It makes them feel fantastic. For example, my client Shirleen Dubuque is fifty-three years old. She loves lifting weights at a very high level of intensity and feeling sore afterward. Another client, Kim Gilhool, is two years younger than Shirleen and can't stand exercise. "I don't like working out, but I do it because I know the alternative is not the best thing," she says.

Though Kim and Shirleen have different attitudes toward exercise, they share the goal of weight loss. You might assume that Shirleen, who loves working out, will lose far more weight than Kim, who can't stand it. You would be wrong. Shirleen has the edge over Kim when it comes to strength, agility, and endurance. However, Kim is only a few steps behind Shirleen when it comes to weight.

Both Shirleen and Kim realized that they would achieve the results they wanted only once they traded unhealthy habits for healthy ones. Imagine a set of dominos lined up one after another. If you knock one domino down in the direction of the other dominos, they all fall down. Your body works the same way. If you lose mental strength, you will lose spiritual strength. If you lose spiritual strength, you will lose emotional strength. If you lose emotional strength, you will lose physical strength. Everything is connected.

MEASURING FITNESS

Some measure physical fitness by how much weight you can bench-press. Others focus on body fat, speed, stamina, or resting heart rate. The truth is, there's no single way to measure fitness. It comes down to lifestyle, sport, job description, body type, muscle length, and even environment. No matter who you are or what you do, fitness means the ability to maintain peak performance. Although proper nutrition is 80 percent of fitness, exercise is also vitally important.

Most folks start exercise programs with goals in mind. Common goals include weight loss, increased muscle mass, completing a marathon, or beating up the bully who made your life miserable in high school. Others exercise because their doctors threaten dire consequences if they don't. Whatever the motivation, they all want to see results as quickly as possible. The fitness industry knows this, which is why most pitches for fitness products and programs promise immediate results.

All those quick-fix health solutions would be bad enough if they simply illustrated our national tendency to value instant gratification over long-term planning and hard work. In fact, they also spread false and pernicious ideas about what it actually takes to get fit.

Case in point: You open a magazine or turn on your television. Up pops a fake doctor touting the latest diet pill, or some guy with abs ripped up like a parking ticket telling you to buy that shiny new exercise machine. Left unsaid is that these characters have probably never used the products they recommend. They're just actors who got paid to say that the pill or gizmo changed their lives and will change your life, too, for just $9.99 a month if you call *right now* for overnight delivery with a full money-back guarantee if not completely satisfied!

Because they're required to by law, these companies also warn you about possible side effects from using their products, such as heart attack, loss of sex drive, nausea, depression, and sudden, agonizing death. But somehow they still manage to make a profit from everyday consumers like you. What's wrong with that picture? If I told you that I smoked and drank alcohol every hour, on the hour, would you still hire me as your fitness coach? I would think not. So why would you pay money for a box of pills that might kill you, or for an exercise gadget that's probably going to wind up gathering dust under your bed? Here's the answer, in two words:

FITNESS ANXIETY

Walk into any gym in America and you're sure to see rows of worried-looking folks, cranking their workout machines like a bunch of neurotic hamsters. Many of them suffer from fitness anxiety. Do you? Here are the symptoms:

- You can't wait to get results.
- You'll do anything to reach your fitness goals, no matter how unhealthy or dangerous it is.
- You get extremely depressed by the numbers on the scale.
- You aren't very good at setting realistic goals.

Though fitness anxiety afflicts both sexes, it's more prevalent among women, who obviously face particular pressure to meet society's standards for physical appearance. Yet men don't get a free pass. Your level of fitness can determine if you get the job or not. It affects work, friendships, and romantic relationships. It's tough to make your colleagues, friends, or spouse happy if you don't feel good about yourself.

Fitness anxiety also drives our national obsession with fad diets, which of course create the infamous yo-yo effect, where you drop weight fast but then gain it all back again after the diet is done. It also drives folks to the gym 7 days a week, hoping to lose weight even faster.

Here's the bad news: Too much exercise can be bad for you. You can actually slow your metabolism by overtraining your body without giving it enough time to rest and recover between workouts. You can also cause serious damage to your tendons, which connect muscle to bone, and your ligaments, which connect bone to bone.

Bottom line: You can't lose weight and get fit overnight. It took some time to stack on the unwanted pounds, and it will take time to get rid of them the right way. I know you want to see results quickly. But you can't rush your body if you want those results to be both positive and lasting. Instead, you need to eat right, exercise, and get plenty of rest. You must cultivate a determined mind and a serene spirit. You must treat your body like it's the only one you've got. As a matter of fact, it is. So make sure to treat it the best you know how.

SHORT AND SWEET

Here's a question I get all the time: "Do I have to train an hour every day to get results?" I don't know what genius made up that rule, but I can tell you that he or she is totally wrong. In my experience, 20 minutes of intense exercise per day can produce results as good as or better than those you'd get from a 1-hour workout, with less wear and tear on your body.

University of Copenhagen researchers recently studied sixty "moderately overweight" Danish men who all wanted to lose weight and committed to regular exercise for 3 months. They separated the chubby Danes into two equal groups. Over the next 3 months, members of the first group ran, biked, and rowed for 60 minutes a day, 7 days a week. The second group worked out daily for 30 minutes. After 3 months, members of the second group had lost an average of 8 pounds, while their peers who worked out twice as long lost only 6 pounds on average.

The study authors reckon that the 30-minute group lost more weight because they had more energy for additional physical exercise after the daily workout. It's also likely that the 60-minute group ate more food and lost less weight as a result. (Some of the difference was probably also due to increased muscle mass.)

Bottom line: There's no need to overdo anything. Training for 1 hour or 2 hours won't give you better results. It simply guarantees that you'll feel really tired the next day. You're better off spending no more than 20 minutes a day in the gym, 5 days a week. Go hard for those 20 minutes. For the rest of the week, focus on nutrition, getting enough rest, and getting your head right by building up your spiritual and mental strength.

That 1-hour-or-nothing attitude can seriously hinder your progress, for real. I can't tell you how many folks I've seen drop out of fitness programs because they didn't think they had enough time to work out. Now, don't get me wrong: If you're a competitive athlete looking to advance in your sport, you'll need to work out much more than the average person. Michael Phelps didn't win twenty-two Olympic medals by spending 20 minutes a day in the pool. However, if your goal is simply to improve your physical appearance and overall health by reducing body fat and increasing muscle, then 20 minutes a day is all you need.

BECOMING AN ATHLETE

The dictionary defines "athlete" as a person who is trained or naturally skilled in games or sports requiring strength, agility, and stamina. I don't agree with this definition at all. For me, an athlete is anyone who is willing to go the extra mile to reach their fitness goals. Here's the key: Athletes never use words like "failure" or "I quit."

This program will challenge you on a mental and physical level. You will feel like giving up at some point. But the minute you start the program, you automatically become an athlete. You do not have to be the strongest or the fastest to take part in this program. All you need is an athletic state of mind.

By that definition, Tricia Rosen is probably the most athletic client I've ever had. Tricia had already faced her share of challenges when we first started working out together. In her early forties, she was a cancer survivor who had recently been in a major car accident that nearly killed her. She was feeling a lot of pain in her spine, shoulders, and ankles that prevented her from living a normal life. On top of that, Tricia had recently buried her mother, who died after a long illness. One of her best friends was dying of cancer, and every week Tricia would help her record an audio diary to leave for her young daughters.

Tricia was a friendly, happy person, a loving mom, and a committed animal rights advocate. Her initial goal was to lose 15 pounds, so I put her on a strict weight-training program. During one of our early workouts we were doing some weight exercises and functional drills that imitated everyday activities like carrying groceries and walking upstairs. About 10 minutes into the workout, Tricia abruptly burst into tears. I still don't know why she was upset, because I never asked her.

"You're here to work out," I said. "Whatever you're feeling, take that energy and put it into the weights."

Tricia looked at me. "Are you serious?" she asked.

"I'm very serious," I replied. Sure enough, she completed the workout, went home smiling, and came back for more.

Ten months into the program, Tricia had already achieved striking results. When she started the program she couldn't do a single pull-up. Now she can do 10 pull-ups. She can bench-press 110 pounds, up from 60 pounds at the beginning of her training. Tricia once struggled to lift 10-pound dumbbells, but now she curls 25-pounders with ease. Most impressive of all, Tricia recently completed her first Tough Mudder 10K race.

Tricia is the female Donovan. She never gives up, just like I never give up. Whatever the barrier in front of her, she'll figure out a way to move that barrier. When Tricia went skiing, she took a fall and broke her tailbone. Most people would be laid up in the hospital with an injury like that. Not Tricia. She called me 2 days after the accident, wanting to work out. No matter how many times I told her no, she insisted on coming to the gym. I modified her exercises so that she was never sitting or lying down, but we still went hard.

Another time she messed up her ankle. The doctors wanted to do surgery, and she showed up at the gym with her foot in a boot. We did all the exercises sitting or lying down: arms, shoulders, legs, back muscles, everything. No matter what life throws at Tricia, she keeps smiling, she keeps working out, and she keeps on moving.

You need that spirit to succeed in any endeavor, including the No Excuses program. Whenever you watch a marathon, you will more than likely think everyone in that marathon is a great runner. In fact, marathons are about completion, not winning. Anyone can enter a marathon and come out a winner simply by finishing the race.

The No Excuses program is based on the start-to-finish principle. I don't accept the words "I can't." All I want to hear is *I can*! There is no room for weakness in this program. Show me a quitter and I will show you a loser. Don't waste your time or mine if you know you are going to quit before you even start.

As they say, practice makes perfect. The more you do something, the better you will become. Athletes who practice their craft improve steadily. The ones who just sit down on their lazy asses become exactly that, lazy asses. It is up to you to either listen or get upset and close this book. If you choose to read further, then I must congratulate you on becoming a true athlete.

FIVE STEPS TO PHYSICAL FITNESS

Here are five steps you should take before embarking on any fitness program, including this one:

1. **Define your goals.**
   Take a few seconds to look at yourself and decide what you want to accomplish. Do you want to gain muscle, lose weight, increase stamina, or just look great in and out of clothing? Please allow me to compare your body to a road trip. You can't take a road trip without mapping out your route. You will never get to your destination if you fail to plan.
2. **Choose relevant exercises.**
   You can't go to law school to become a doctor; you will have to go to medical school to achieve that goal. Knowing the type of training needed to meet your

specific needs is just as critical. If you want to become more flexible, then weight training is not your best choice. Instead choose something like yoga or Pilates. Also, don't waste time following what other people are doing. Stick to your own plan.

3. **Stay committed.**

   Quitting is easy. Many people drop out of their fitness program before gaining any results. Your body will not change in a couple of months. Expecting change this fast is like putting fresh paint on a wall and pressing your back against it immediately. What a mess! Instead, start by setting short- and long-term goals. Be patient and do not quit. Keep your muscles happy by constantly training both mind and body. Avoid excuses and get your butt to the gym.

4. **Lift weights.**

   Cardio 2 to 3 days per week is great, and everyone needs to stay limber by following a stretching regime. However, you should also lift weights no matter what your fitness goals are. Weight training is the peanut butter to a sandwich. Lifting weights will help to burn extra calories while keeping your bones strong and your confidence high. You should lift weights that are heavy enough to force your muscles to contract (squeeze). Include calisthenics exercises such as push-ups, pull-ups, dips, and sprints in your regimen. You will not be disappointed.

5. **Eat clean.**

   Even if you own the world's most expensive car, no fuel means no go. Going to the gym and running outdoors are great for your body and mind. However, proper nourishment is crucial to building and toning your body. You have to fuel your body properly all day. Avoid processed foods and drink lots of water. Eat minimum amounts of simple sugars and always include proteins, carbohydrates, and fats in each meal.

You must follow these basic guidelines to become a stronger and better you. Keep an open mind and don't let anyone or anything stop you from reaching your goals.

GYM OR HOME?

Where you train comes down to personal preference. Physically speaking, there's nothing you can do in the gym that you can't do at home, with a little imagination. Still, working out at home is undeniably a different experience compared to hitting the gym, so let's weigh up some of the pluses and minuses in both environments.

Gyms offer sophisticated equipment and other patrons who either share your goals or have already achieved them. The level of motivation is extremely high, especially if you pick a gym frequented by great-looking people. Gyms also boast personal trainers who can help you optimize your workout and avoid injury. Finally, your home likely doesn't offer fitness classes, saunas, and juice bars.

On the downside, you'll probably have to commit to your gym for a year or so, although in these tough economic times many gyms have started rethinking the contract requirement. Going to the gym also takes more time than working out at home. Beyond the actual workout, you have to deal with traffic and parking, not to mention parking tickets.

Okay, so you finally get inside the gym after dealing with all that ruckus and now you have to face the after-work crowd that just swarmed in like a colony of anxious bees. There are no machines available, and some freakishly muscular dude in spandex is hogging the bench press. All this can be very annoying, to the point where you just want to go home and work out another day. More than likely, that day will never come.

Alternatively, you can work out at home. Your home gym probably won't have high-tech equipment or a crowd of folks to motivate you. It does offer privacy, with nobody watching or judging you. I personally enjoy exercising at home. I visit my local gym once or twice a month, but I'm at home for the most part. I work out in the basement of my house, where I've rigged up a simple gym that consists of barbells, dumbbells, punching bag, squat rack, functional trainer, medicine ball, jump rope, stepper, kettle bells, and exercise mat. I bought everything used, and the entire setup cost me less than $1,000. (You can get started for less than $100—see the box below.) I don't worry about paying gym membership or babysitting fees or even getting a parking ticket. I just roll out of bed, walk down the stairs, and *boom*, I'm working out!

HOW TO BUILD A HOME GYM FOR LESS THAN $100

Your local gym might boast fancy workout machines and a gourmet juice bar, but you can outfit an excellent home gym for less than the monthly cost of a typical gym membership. All these items are available online, at specialized fitness stores, or in the fitness section of your local department store.

Item	Approximate Cost
1 jump rope	$5
1 exercise/yoga mat	$10
1 pair 10-pound dumbbells	$20
1 medium-weight resistance band	$12
1 pair push-up bars	$15
1 medicine ball (8 pounds)	$20
1 large inflatable balancing ball	$15
TOTAL	$97

SEVEN STEPS TO SUCCESS

Here are seven key steps to achieving your fitness goals:

1. **Train just enough.**

   Though exercise is great, it's not a good idea to work out every single day of the week. Excessive training won't yield faster results. On the contrary, it will set you up for a frustrating plateau and allow new problems to slip in, among them fatigue, weight gain, loss of mental focus, and muscle atrophy. For optimal results, train 5 days per week and rest the other 2 days.

2. **Set realistic goals.**

   Your goals must be attainable, time bound, and enjoyable. If you set out to pump iron for 3 hours every day after several years of inactivity, you are setting yourself up for failure, not to mention injury. Start by working out for 20 minutes a day, following the workout schedule in Chapter 7. Allow for the inevitable setbacks, like that irresistible slice of birthday cake or the day when you skip a workout because your child is sick or you have to deal with a crisis at work.

3. **Train nice and slow at first.**

   Don't think you are not making progress unless you train like a Navy SEAL on steroids. Excessive training yields extreme muscle soreness, which will deter you from going back to the gym. Start off nice and slow and train like a beginner. Take the time to learn proper form. Don't work out with a friend who's ahead of you in training. He or she will expect you to keep up, and you will only hurt yourself. There is a good kind of sore and a bad kind; you'll know the difference as you advance in your fitness regime.

4. **Catch your z's.**

   Make sure you get 6 to 8 hours of sleep every day. You must allow your body to recharge so that you have enough energy to perform on a day-to-day basis. If you don't get enough sleep, you'll diminish proper brain function and the ability to think clearly. You will also reduce your body's ability to burn fat the way it needs to.

5. **Drink water.**

   Water should be the first thing you drink when you wake up in the morning and the last thing you drink before going to sleep. Water transports nutrients throughout your body. You need it to keep your organs fully functional, and it also helps to regulate body temperature. All you have to do is look at plants that haven't been watered enough. You'll look the same way if you don't drink enough water.

6. **Keep moving.**

   We all start off strong but eventually lose the motivation to continue. You must find ways to reboot your motivation. Look at pictures of yourself before you gained weight, or of someone else whose physique inspires you. Program your phone calendar so it prompts you to eat right, exercise, and drink your water. Getting family and friends involved is another great way to stay motivated. Give them the responsibility of keeping you on track by calling, texting, or e-mailing you to remind you to stay on track. And make sure to pick exercises that you enjoy. If your workout isn't fun, you'll drift.

7. **Prioritize fitness.**

   Many Americans start pursuing a fitness program when the doctor tells them it's a matter of life and death. It's sad that only bad news can be such a powerful motivator. But you don't have to wait.

KNOW YOUR BODY

How well do you know yourself? Before you start this program, note down your weight and your body-fat percentage. Measure your waist, thighs, hips, stomach, arms, chest, and neck. If you can squeeze a metabolic test into your budget, so much the better. This test will tell you how many calories your body burns when it's at rest.

You should make a list of the things that make you happy, as well as those that make you angry. As you learn more about yourself, you will realize that you are solely responsible for your successes and your failures. Nobody can force you to do what you don't want to do. You'll make mistakes along the way, but mistakes don't mean the end of the road. They mean you're human. So when you fall down and get dirty, just pick yourself up and keep moving.

And remember: *You can do this!*

CHAPTER 7

The No Excuses Program

Congratulations! Your life is about to change. You are embarking on a 30-day fitness journey divided into three equal phases: Think, Reach, and Move. I designed the three phases to track a steady progression from a sedentary lifestyle to an active, healthy one. Much like the martial arts, the No Excuses program is a progressive system in which you rise through a series of levels as your flexibility, strength, and stamina improve.

I set weight-loss and attitude-readjustment goals for each of the three phases. If you follow the program diligently, you can expect to lose 10 pounds over the 30 days. More important, you'll emerge with the mental strength and serenity to make wise health and nutrition choices going forward, which will ensure that you keep the weight off and meet your personal wellness goals.

Think about how you feel when you wake up in the morning. Before you're ready to face the new day, you need to take a shower, brush your teeth, get dressed, put on your perfume or cologne, and hopefully eat your breakfast. Once that sequence is complete, you're ready to take on the world. You feel so fresh and clean that it's almost a shame to get dirty all over again.

Fitness programs, similarly, are all about mental and physical preparation. You should constantly remind yourself of your short- and long-term goals. Log your daily activities, including meals, workouts, thoughts, and emotions. Allow yourself a treat when you do great, like a movie outing or a new pair of jeans. You should also impose restrictions on yourself when you backslide, such as no TV or sweets for a week.

I know that you're an adult, not a child. But guess what: Kids aren't the only ones who respond well to boundaries, clear goals, and a system of rewards for good behavior and penalties for bad. Learn how to bring out your inner child and have some fun with the process. You might be surprised by the outcome.

I'm very excited to get you started on this program, and I know you are too. I will speak in a simple, clear, and realistic manner, with no scientific or technical jargon. Please understand, however, that I won't speak to you with a soft tone. As I tell my clients: We're here to work out. I understand that life sometimes gets in the way of our goals, but I'm not interested in hearing excuses.

There are many possible barriers to creating and completing a healthy and successful fitness program. They can include job and child-care responsibilities, relationship issues, or simply lack of motivation. No matter what your situation is, you can't let life's pressures kill your focus. Before you venture into the world of fitness, you must ensure that you are mentally and physically prepared for the journey.

This is the beginning of your new life, and I want it to be almost perfect. I say "almost," because nothing in this world is really perfect; there is always a flaw. But almost perfect is good enough.

PHASE ONE: THINK

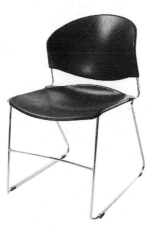

In the Think phase of my No Excuses program we're going to concentrate on getting your mind right. I'll start you off on a mental cleanse that's designed to help you manage stress and stay focused on your goals. I'll give you a specific task to complete every day. These tasks range from simple steps like purging your refrigerator of junk food to more demanding ones like creating a home gym, spending quality time with your family, and reviving old friendships.

A cleanse is one of the most important things you can do before you try to lose weight, build muscle, lose body fat, or get faster. It's like spring cleaning, when you get rid of the old and make room for the new. You might eat a healthy diet and exercise 7 days a week. None of it will matter if your stress levels are high and you don't feel good about yourself. Even if you are happy now, there is always room for more happiness.

Every day I'll give you a specific mental mission to complete. Your job is to complete each day's mission and write down how you felt after each completion. Don't forget to keep track of your emotions. If you felt sad, happy, angry, horny, drunk, or amused, just write it down. Don't skip any days at all. Good luck: Your life change begins now.

On the physical side, I believe that nutrition and flexibility are essential to mental clarity and peace. A poor diet and a stiff body will collude to inflict stress on your mind. During the Think phase you'll practice a daily stretching-and-strength regime based on movements from yoga and sports conditioning. The exercises in the Think phase of the No Excuses program are based on my popular "Healthy Couch Potato" series of video workouts, featured on *The Dr. Oz Show* website. They are designed as a fitness on-ramp for sedentary readers, which is why every Think exercise can be performed while sitting on a couch.

You need only 20 minutes of No Excuses training a day to look and feel your best. I need to warn you, however, that my workouts will challenge your body and mind to the utmost. Muscles respond best when you train them continuously, with minimal rest. Continuous training forces your muscles to burn maximum energy, which in turn stimulates the fat-burning process throughout your body. That's why No Excuses workouts incorporate circuit training, where you go from one exercise to the next with little or no rest after each completed set.

The human body can take a lot more stress than most of us put it through. If you go to the gym and watch the average person working out, you'll see that they spend more time resting and talking than they do exercising. If you want exceptional results, you must push your body to the point of pure muscular failure, where even your nervous system goes on the fritz. That doesn't mean you have to overtrain: Again, I'm asking you to work out only 20 minutes a day. In those 20 minutes, however, you must push your mind to push your body.

Note: No specific exercise below is better than any other. I am giving you a total-body workout that requires each move to be executed properly. Always maintain proper form, and avoid movements that could aggravate an old injury. Before you embark on this training program, make sure to get full clearance from your physician.

Let's begin!

THINK DAY 1

Welcome to the No Excuses program! When you wake up, go straight to your kitchen, pour yourself a glass of room-temperature water, and squeeze into it juice from ½ lemon. (Avoid cold water, which will unduly shock your organs first thing in the morning.) Drink it before you do anything else. When the glass is empty, pull out your juicer and treat yourself to a Caribbean Eye Opener (recipe on page 163).

Mental Exercise: What Makes You Happy?

It's time to start taking care of your head. Stand in front of a mirror for 1 minute. Breathe in deeply through your nose and out through your mouth (about 15 breaths). Think about what makes you happy. I want you to return to this exercise throughout the day. Whenever you have a minute to spare, just breathe and concentrate on something that lifts your spirits. It could be a loved one, a happy memory, or an experience that you're looking forward to. For me it's my children.

NUTRITION TIP #1

Every morning when you wake up, drink a glass of lukewarm water with the juice of ½ lemon. Lemon juice improves intestinal function, which will help burn belly fat.

MENTAL CLEANSE #1

Starting today, keep a daily journal. Make sure to log your meals, your workouts, and your state of mind.

Okay, now go shower and get dressed. It's time for breakfast! I recommend my Funky Kingston Smoothie, or any of the delicious recipes in Chapter 8. Wait at least 30 minutes before proceeding to the next step, which is your first workout in the No Excuses program.

Workout: Seated Power

Goal: General flexibility and strength

Are you ready? Let's go. If you, like most people, have been sedentary for a while, let's start with a simple stretching-and-strength routine that you can perform while seated on a couch or chair. Any kind of surface is fine, but firmer is better. And don't get too relaxed: Just because you're sitting down doesn't mean you won't be working hard.

The goal of this entire program is to help you supercharge your health and ditch what drags you down. Sometimes we all feel like we're in jail, so think of these exercises as a jailbreak. Like every workout in this book, the goal is to raise your heartbeat and keep it raised for 20 minutes. Do every exercise for the specified time and then move to the next one immediately, with as little rest as possible. When you're done with all 10 exercises, go back to the beginning and keep cycling through the exercises for 20 minutes. Don't forget to breathe during each exercise, and take a short water break every 5 to 6 minutes during your workout.

Note: To minimize the risk of injury, it's vital that you warm up and stretch your muscles before and after every workout. You'll find a simple stretching regime on page 193.

SEATED JUMPING JACKS

Just like regular jumping jacks, except you're sitting down.

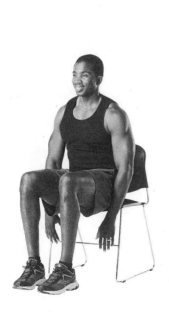
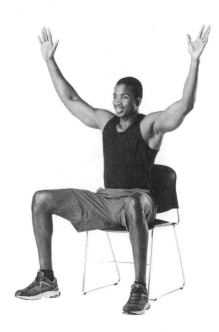

SEATED SCISSOR SWITCH

Place your hands behind your head, keeping your back straight and your chin up. Move one foot forward and the other foot back. Repeat for 60 seconds, alternating the forward foot.

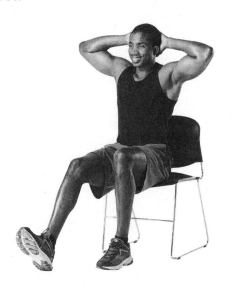
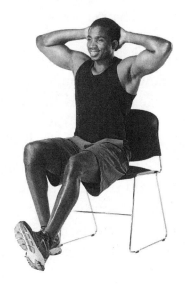

SEATED FEET IN, FEET OUT

Start in a seated position, back straight, hands in fighting stance, feet together. Hop both feet forward, then pull them back in. Repeat for 60 seconds.

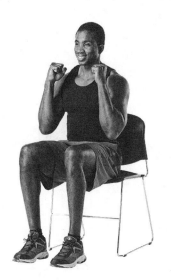
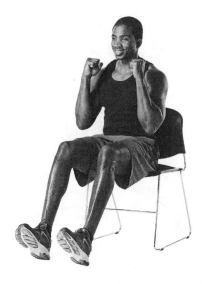

SEATED WIDE LEG STRETCH

Spread your legs apart as far as they will go. Reach forward, keeping your back straight, and touch the ground. Return to starting position and repeat.

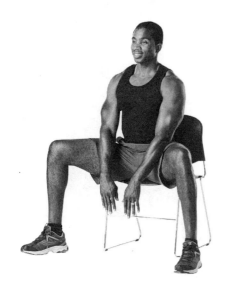 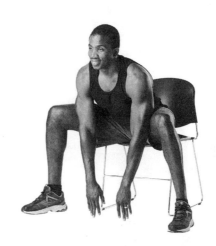

SEATED HAMSTRING STRETCH

Extend your right leg and flex your ankle so that your toes are pointed toward you. Reach as far as you can down your leg. Hold for 15 seconds. Repeat with your left leg.

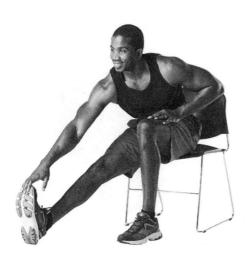 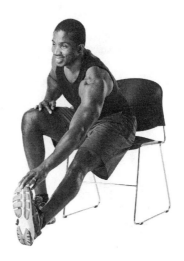

SEATED REACH FOR THE STARS

Extend your arms above your head, lace your fingers together, and hold for 30 seconds.

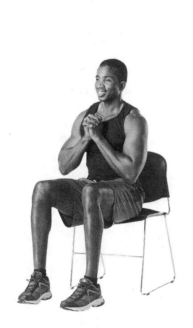
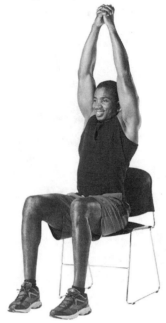

SEATED ALTERNATING REACH AND TOUCH

From a seated position, reach down and touch your left foot with your right hand. Return to an upright seated position. Reach down and touch your right foot with your left hand. Continue for 30 seconds, alternating sides.

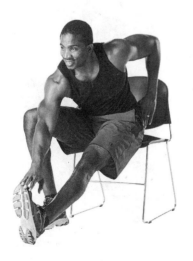
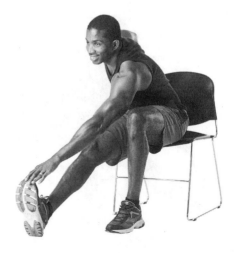

SEATED JOG IN PLACE

From a seated position, move your feet like you're jogging. Go as fast as you can for 30 seconds.

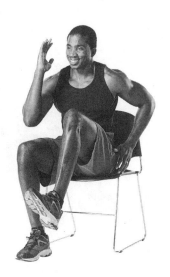 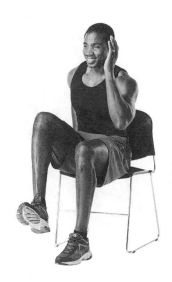

SEATED OBLIQUE TWISTS

Sit upright toward the edge of your seat. Rotate your trunk left and right, holding your fists up like you're about to fight.

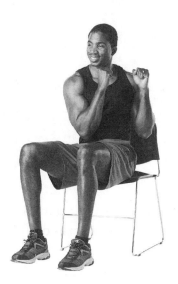 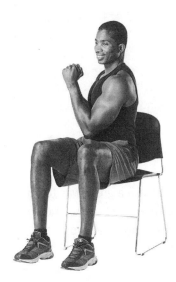

SEATED FRONT STRETCH

Extend both legs straight out in front of you. Reach out and grab the toes of your right foot with your left hand. If you can't reach your toes, no problem. Just move your hand as far down your leg as you can to get a good stretch. Repeat, alternating sides.

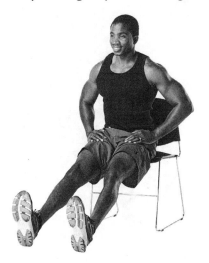 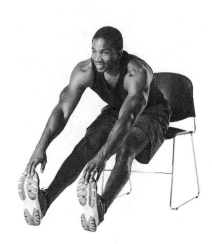

THINK DAY 2

NUTRITION TIP #2

Add 2 tablespoons of flaxseed to your oatmeal or smoothie. Flaxseed will boost your intake of healthy fiber and omega-3 fatty acids.

MENTAL CLEANSE #2

Don't forget to take deep breaths in and out throughout the day. Conscious breathing is a form of meditation and a great reminder that you're alive.

MYTHBUSTER

Myth: Crunches are a great way to flatten your stomach.
Fact: A flat stomach actually comes from eating foods that are low in fat and refined sugars. No matter how many crunches you do, they will build only the muscle that lies deep beneath those unforgiving layers of fat.

Workout: Free Your Shoulders

Goal: Increase shoulder strength and mobility

Many people struggle with mobility in their shoulders due to lack of flexibility and range of motion. And many of us get shoulder injuries from daily activities, like steering a car, lugging a kid around, and hefting bags of groceries. The goal of this workout is to increase range of motion and flexibility in your shoulders so you can get through all your daily activities with minimal stress and pain.

SHOULDER ROTATIONS

Extend your arms straight out in front of you, palms down (pronated). Rotate your arms outward so your palms are up (supinated). Squeeze your chest muscles while rotating. Repeat for 60 seconds.

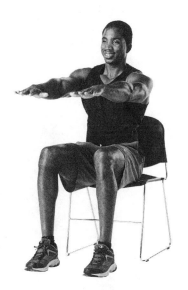 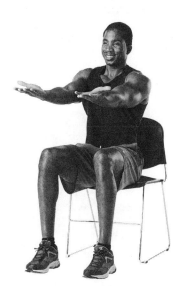

THIS IS A STICKUP

Sit straight up and keep your back straight. Raise your arms, elbows bent 90 degrees, triceps parallel to floor, palms facing forward. Extend your arms straight above your head. Imagine I've got a gun and this is a stickup. Come back down to the starting position. Repeat for 60 seconds.

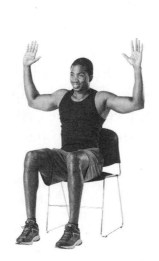
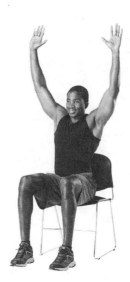

THUNDERCLAP

Extend your arms straight out to your sides, fingers separated, palms out. Bring your arms in together until your palms meet in a clap, keeping your fingers separated. Repeat for 60 seconds.

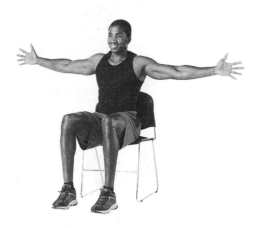
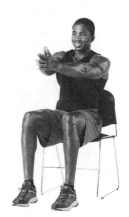

ZOMBIE SHOULDER FLUTTER

Start with your arms straight out in front of you, shoulder width apart, palms down, like a zombie marching through the night. Lift your left arm up while bringing your right arm down. Repeat as fast as you can, alternating arms for 60 seconds.

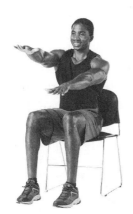
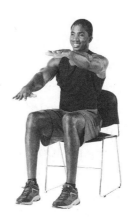

JAILBREAK

Imagine you're climbing up a perimeter fence and busting out of jail. Start sitting, with vertical posture, your back straight. Raise your left arm straight up, palm out, like you're reaching for a handhold. Your right arm is bent, palm forward at shoulder height. Alternate raising and lowering your arms as quickly as possible. Picture a spotlight on your back and guards aiming to shoot you the hell up. Repeat for 60 seconds.

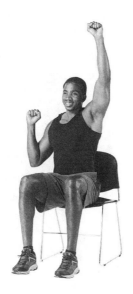
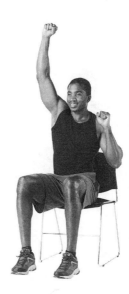

GREAT JOB, SKIPPY!

Scoot your butt to the edge of your seat if you are seated. Extend your arms, elbows bent, palms underneath your thighs, both thumbs up (like you're saying "good job"), feet together. Leaning forward so your body is at a 45-degree angle, pull your arms back, thumbs pointing toward the back, squeezing your shoulder blades together. Return to the starting position, and repeat for 60 seconds.

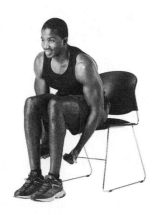 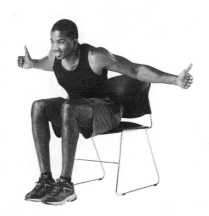

MICHAEL SCARECROW

Michael Jackson used this move when he played the Scarecrow in *The Wiz*. Sit at the edge of your seat with your back straight, your arms raised, and your elbows bent at 90 degrees. Rotate your shoulders by dropping your palms down like a scarecrow. Keep your triceps parallel to the floor, and go as far as you can without rounding your chest or your back. Repeat for 60 seconds.

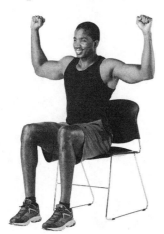 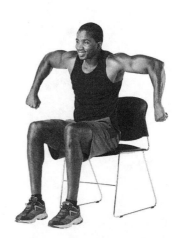

TOUCHDOWN

Begin with your arms down, palms facing you. Extend your arms all the way out to your sides, palms down and parallel to the floor. Raise your arms above your head, rotating your palms inward, keeping your biceps aligned with your ears. Finish with your arms straight above your head, palms facing inward, like a football referee calling a touchdown. The goal is to keep your arms straight throughout the exercise. As your flexibility and range of motion improve, you'll be able to bring your palms closer and closer together. The ultimate goal is to be able to touch your palms together with your arms straight above your head. Repeat for 60 seconds.

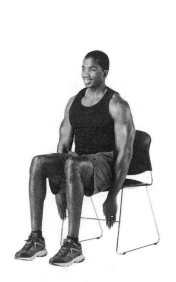 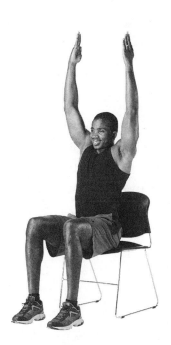

I DON'T KNOW

Perch on the edge of your seat, with your back straight and your posture vertical. Drop your arms to your sides, relaxing your shoulders but keeping your stomach tight and your chest lifted. Raise your shoulders as high as you can toward your ears, return to the starting position, then repeat for 60 seconds. It's like saying "I don't know" with some attitude, over and over.

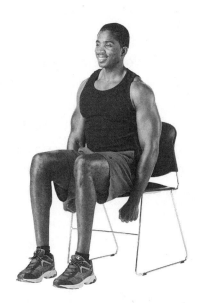 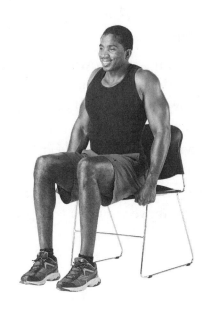

ACCORDION SQUEEZE

Perch on the edge of your seat, with your back straight and your posture vertical. Bend your elbows at 90 degrees and pull your shoulders back. Turn your palms inward and make two tight fists. Keeping your upper arms locked at your sides, rotate your forearms backward and then forward to the starting position, like you're playing the accordion in a polka band. *Prost!*

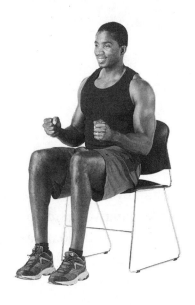 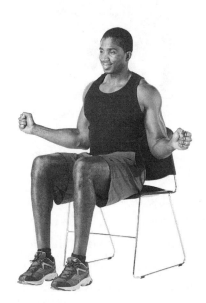

THINK DAY 3

NUTRITION TIP #3

Add more vegetables to your meals, preferably leafy green ones like kale, spinach, and bok choy. Green veggies are a great source of vitamins and minerals and will help keep your organs and muscles in tip-top shape.

MENTAL CLEANSE #3

Make a to-do list of things you failed to accomplish in the past. Do them one by one, starting today.

MYTHBUSTER

Myth: I don't need to warm up before exercise.
Fact: A proper warm-up will help prevent injuries to cold, tight muscles. Warming up also puts your body and mind in the proper state for exercise. Jumping jacks are a great way to warm up, and so are stretches. You'll find a full-body stretching routine on page 193.

Workout: Show Some Leg

Goal: Strengthen leg muscles

Your legs are your foundation. The stronger the foundation, the stronger the house. This workout builds foundational strength in your primary leg muscles, including the gluteus maximus (butt), quadriceps (front thigh), hamstrings (back of thighs), gastrocnemius (calf muscles), adductors (inner thigh), and abductors (outer thigh).

Note: Begin every exercise in this workout by sitting toward the edge of your seat, with your knees bent at 90 degrees. Your ankles should be aligned with your knees. Keep your back straight and your posture vertical.

DRACULA KICK

Cross your arms over your chest like Dracula in his coffin. Keep your right leg bent at 90 degrees, your ankle aligned with your knee. Extend your left leg fully forward, and pull your toes in toward your shin. Raise your left leg as high as you can, keeping it straight and contracting your thigh muscles (quadriceps). Repeat for 30 seconds, then switch legs and repeat for another 30 seconds.

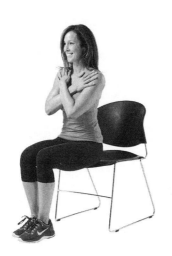 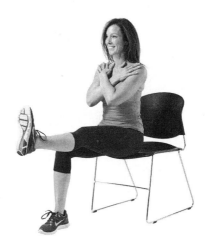

PUPPET MARCH

Raise your left knee and right elbow together. Repeat for 60 seconds, alternating knees and elbows, like you're Pinocchio busting out of the toy store.

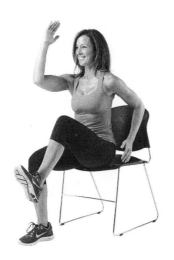 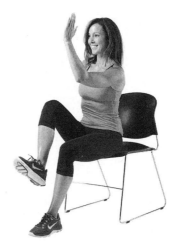

SEATED BABY BOOSTER

Lift your heels off the ground as high as you can while contracting your calf muscles. Touch your heels lightly to the ground and repeat like you're bouncing a baby on your lap. Repeat as fast as you can for 60 seconds. To add more resistance, place your palms on top of your knees and press down firmly as you lift your heels.

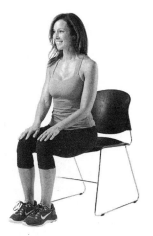 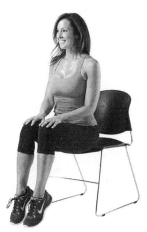

CURFEW VIOLATION

Keeping your knees bent at 90 degrees, raise your left leg as high as you can and swing it out to the side like you're a teenager exiting the house through her bedroom window after curfew. Your right leg follows in the same direction, ending next to your left leg. Next, raise and swing your right leg toward the right and follow with your left leg. Repeat for 60 seconds.

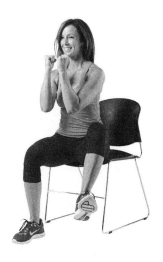 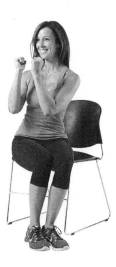

KICK DOWN THE DOOR

Pull your left knee in as far as possible toward your chest. Shrimp up your body by rounding your back so you look like a crustacean. Extend your left leg outward. Keep your toes flexed in toward your shin while opening your chest and straightening your back. Imagine you're a firefighter kicking in a door so you can rescue someone from a burning building. Repeat for 60 seconds, alternating legs.

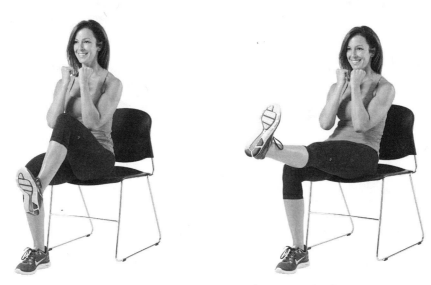

Do four complete sets (or as many as you can) for a total of 20 minutes. Don't forget water breaks!

THINK DAY 4

NUTRITION TIP #4

Avoid store-bought salad dressings, which tend to be very high in fat and sugars. Instead, dress your salad in a little extra-virgin olive oil or lemon juice.

MENTAL CLEANSE #4

Crank your favorite song on the stereo. Dance and sing along. This will get your heart rate up, burn calories, reduce stress, *and* release endorphins, those magic brain chemicals that make you feel happy.

Workout: Range Expander

Goal: Boost flexibility and range of motion

If your muscles are tight and inflexible, your range of motion will be limited, which will hurt your performance both in and out of the gym. The good news is that you can achieve good range of motion without tying your legs behind your head like a master yogi. This workout is designed to increase your natural range of motion. We're hitting the neck, shoulders, hips, ankles, hamstrings, inner thighs, trunk, and lower back. Follow these simple yet effective moves and I guarantee you will see results within a few days.

Note: Start all exercises by perching on the edge of your seat, back straight, and posture vertical.

SHOULDER ROLLS (FORWARD AND BACK)

Drop your arms to your sides, relaxing your shoulders but keeping your stomach tight and your chest lifted. Lift your shoulders as high as possible. Then retract them toward the back, squeezing your shoulder blades together. Return to the starting position and repeat in a circular motion for 30 seconds. Next, reverse the motion by lifting and rotating your shoulders forward, separating your shoulder blades as you move. Repeat for 30 seconds.

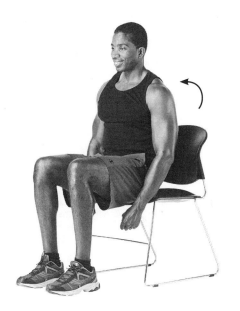 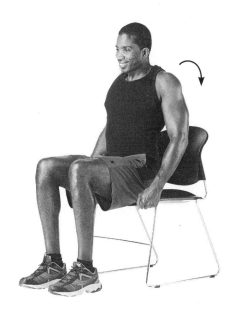

SMALL ARM CIRCLES

Extend your arms out to the sides, with palms facing out and fingers pulled in toward your ears. Make small backward circles for 30 seconds, then small forward circles for another 30 seconds. Raise your left knee as high as you can during the backward circles, and your right knee as high as you can during the forward circles. Trust me, that's a burn, even for me.

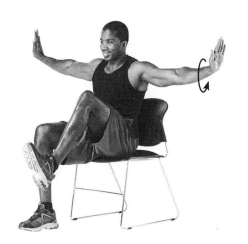 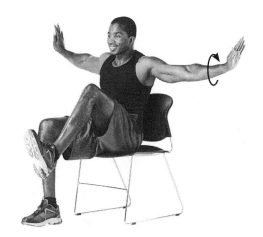

BIG ARM CIRCLES

Use the same starting position and movements as you did in Small Arm Circles, except make bigger circles and keep your feet planted. Repeat for 30 seconds in each direction.

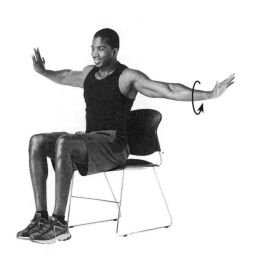 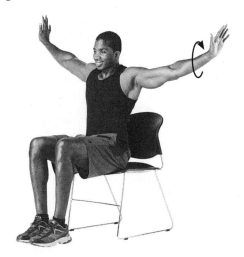

TRUNK FLEXES

Maintaining that ramrod posture, flex your trunk to the right and come back to vertical. Then flex to the left and return to vertical. Keep your arms hanging naturally at your sides. You should feel a good stretch in your waist on the side opposite the stretch, so your right side stretches as your trunk drops to the left and vice versa. Repeat for 60 seconds.

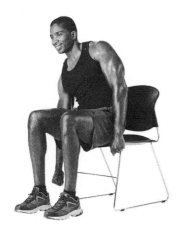 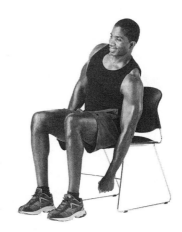

SITTING ALTERNATE KNEE PULL

Grab the front of your left knee with both hands and pull it in toward your chest as far as possible, keeping your back straight and your shoulders dropped. Hold for 5 seconds, then repeat with your right knee and continue alternating knees for 60 seconds.

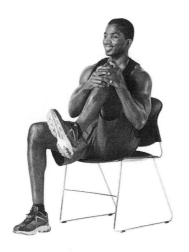 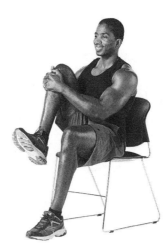

KNEE CIRCLES (BOTH DIRECTIONS)

Lift your left foot about 3 inches off the floor and rotate your lower leg clockwise from the knee, making circles in the air for 30 seconds. Repeat with your left leg counterclockwise, then switch to your right leg and repeat the entire sequence for a total of 2 minutes. Keep your feet parallel to the floor throughout the exercise. This one helps develop range of motion in your knees. It also strengthens your hip muscles. Bonus: It gives your quadriceps a great burn.

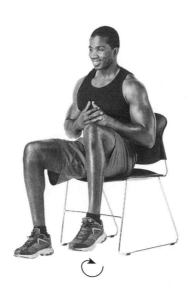

ANKLE ROTATION

Sit back in your seat and extend both your legs fully, lifting your feet off the ground and pulling your toes in toward your shins. Rotate your feet in opposite directions so that your right foot is circulating clockwise while your left foot circulates counterclockwise. Continue for 30 seconds and then reverse the direction of your feet (left foot clockwise, right foot counterclockwise).

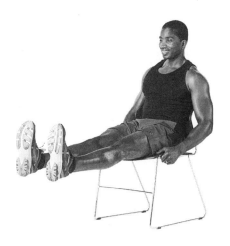
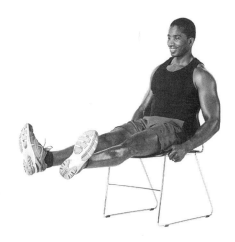

STRAIGHT-LEG HAMSTRING STRETCH

Keeping your legs shoulder width apart, extend them fully in front of you, heels touching the ground and toes pulled in toward your shins. Push your chest forward as you bend from the hips, keeping your back straight. Slide your hands down your legs as far as you can without rounding your back. Hold for 20 seconds, rest for 10 seconds, and repeat once.

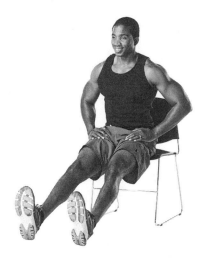
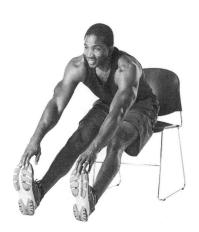

SEATED REACH AND TOUCH

Spread your knees as far as you can past shoulder width. Your arms should hang down between your inner thighs, fingers pointing to the floor. Reach down and touch the floor, bringing your chest parallel to the ground. Place your palms on the floor if you can, or simply touch your fingers to the floor to start with. Return to the starting position and raise your arms straight above your head, palms out. Repeat for 30 seconds.

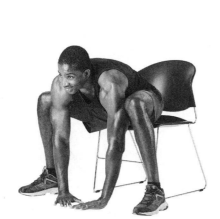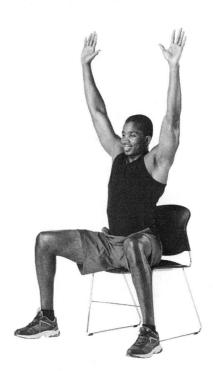

NECK ROTATIONS

Place your hands and forearms on top of your thighs, palms down. Look straight ahead, keeping your chin parallel to the floor. Relax your shoulders and turn your head as far as you can to the left. Try to see as much behind your back as you can, using your peripheral vision. Hold this position for 5 seconds, and then return to the starting position. Repeat on your right side, holding for 5 seconds, and then return to center. Then point your chin upward toward the ceiling, hold for 5 seconds, and return to center. Now look down, bringing your chin toward your chest. Hold for 5 seconds, and return to center. Continue on all sides for total of 60 seconds.

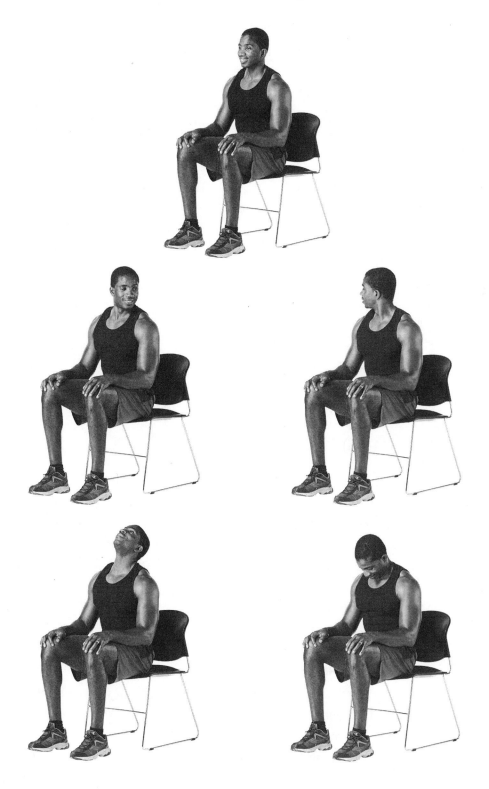

THINK DAY 5

MYTHBUSTER

Myth: Cardio is only for folks who want to lose weight.
Fact: Even Superman needs cardio to stay in tip-top shape. Your heart is your engine, and without a strong engine you'll never get far.

Workout: Seated Cardio Burn

Goal: Build stamina and burn fat

This workout targets your cardiovascular system. The goal is to increase stamina and burn fat without using expensive equipment. As with all Think workouts, you can do every single one of these exercises while sitting on your favorite chair.

Note: Start all exercises sitting at the edge of your seat with vertical posture, feet together, knees bent 90 degrees.

SEATED PUNCH JACKS

Start with your elbows tight to your body and bent at about 90 degrees, hands facing inward, fists tight. Lift your elbows out to the sides, keeping your feet together, then punch straight out, one arm at a time, while separating your legs. Finish with your arms fully extended, fists together, legs spread, and then return to the starting position. Repeat the motion, but this time punch toward the sky while separating your legs. Repeat for 60 seconds, alternating forward and upward punches.

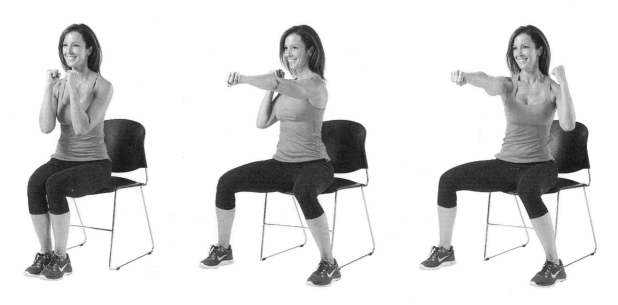

TREASURE CHEST

Raise your arms so that your triceps are parallel to floor. Your elbows should be bent 90 degrees, with your palms facing forward and your fists clenched. Squeeze your elbows together while rotating your palms inward. Pretend you have a gold doubloon clenched between your chest (pectoralis) muscles, like Captain Morgan showing off in a night-club. Repeat as fast as you can for 60 seconds.

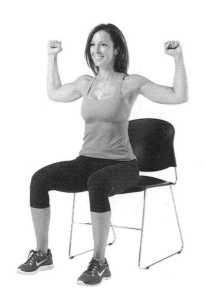
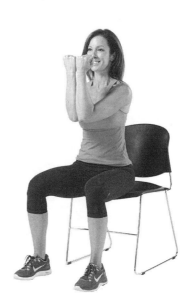

KNEE-TO-ELBOW MARCH

Start with your elbows bent, hands interlaced behind your head. Maintaining straight posture, lift your left leg (keeping your left knee bent) while rotating your right elbow toward your left knee. Repeat on the opposite side (left elbow to right knee). Alternate sides for 60 seconds.

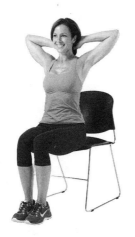 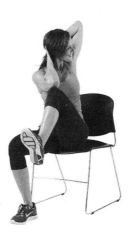

PRISON SIDE BENDS

Keep your hands interlaced behind your head and your elbows out to the sides, squeezing your shoulder blades together. Tighten up your midsection while leaning over to the left so you get a good stretch on your right side (oblique muscles). Repeat for 60 seconds, alternating sides. To increase the cardio burn, shorten up the movements and increase your speed.

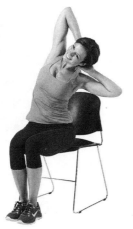 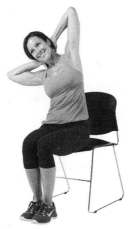

RUMBLE IN THE BRONX

Start with your shoulders relaxed and your fists raised at both sides of your jaw, like you're getting ready for a bar fight. Punch straight out with your left fist, pushing your left shoulder forward while pulling your right shoulder back. Then punch out with your right fist and repeat for 60 seconds, alternating left and right punches as fast as you can.

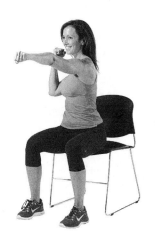 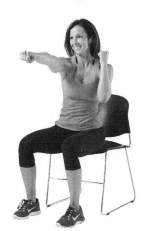

ROCKETTE LEG SWINGS

Last exercise! Keeping your right knee bent at 90 degrees, extend your left leg fully. Lift that leg and trace a high half circle to the left. Then return the leg to the starting position, tracing the same half circle in reverse. Repeat for 60 seconds, then switch legs and repeat for another 60 seconds. Take a bow, 'cause your workout is done!

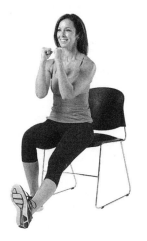 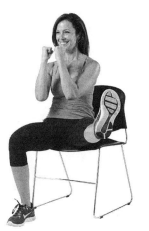 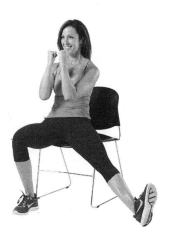

THINK DAY 6

REST DAY!

Do something active but low impact, like a 30-minute walk in the park, holding light dumbbells. Or get a massage. Repeat one of the five Think workouts if you feel like it, or choose one of the Sneak-Attack Workouts starting on page 199.

NUTRITION TIP #6

If you're a coffee drinker, switch to organic coffee. It has more antioxidants to help you fight off cancer-causing cells.

MENTAL CLEANSE #6

Clean out one of your closets. Getting rid of old clothing will give you room for the new stuff, especially when you start slimming down. Put the old clothing to good use by donating it to your local shelter.

MYTHBUSTER

Myth: Walking won't help me lose weight.
Fact: Walking will absolutely help you lose weight, assuming you walk at least 5 times weekly for a minimum of 30 minutes a day. Challenge yourself to walk faster and farther as your body gets used to the exercise.

THINK DAY 7

Workout: Repeat Show Some Leg (Think Day 3, page 85)

Goal: Strengthen leg muscles

NUTRITION TIP #7

Cut down on your salt intake. Instead, flavor your food with fresh herbs and spices, which will help lower your blood pressure. I use a little bit of sea salt in many of my recipes, but much of the flavor comes from spices like basil, oregano, paprika, and cayenne pepper.

MENTAL CLEANSE #7

Make a list of ten people in your life whom you absolutely love. Starting today, call one of them on the phone each day for the next 10 days and tell them how you feel. **Note:** Do not text or e-mail. Pick up the damn phone and call your friends.

MYTHBUSTER

Myth: You can lose fat from specific parts of your body by exercising those spots.
Fact: There are no shortcuts to fat loss. If you do full-body strength training and cardio workouts, the excess fat will eventually come off from the places where you want it gone.

THINK DAY 8

Workout: Repeat Seated Power (Think Day 1, page 73)

Goal: General flexibility and strength

NUTRITION TIP #8

Take vitamins D and C, following the recommended dosage for your age. Vitamin D is essential for bone strength, and vitamin C will help strengthen your immune system.

MENTAL CLEANSE #8

Open up a special savings account to reward yourself for getting fit. Deposit small sums whenever you can, nothing crazy. I deposit anywhere between $1 and $5 at a time in my savings account, which I call "Fit Fun." I build up the balance for about 3 months and then use the money to pay for new sneakers, take my kids out for ice cream, or help to pay for a family vacation—just whatever comes up and makes me feel good.

MYTHBUSTER

Myth: The more you sweat during exercise, the more fat you lose.
Fact: The harder you work out, the more calories you'll burn within a given period. But how much you sweat has nothing to do with how much fat you lose.

THINK DAY 9

Workout: Repeat Seated Cardio Burn (Think Day 5, page 96)

Goal: Build stamina and burn fat

NUTRITION TIP #9

Eat every 2 to 3 hours. This will boost your metabolism and prevent your body from storing unnecessary fat.

MENTAL CLEANSE #9

Clean your house with natural products that spread a calming aroma throughout your home. A good-smelling house will help you build a healthy spirit. A clean home will also help you to think more clearly, without feeling cluttered.

MYTHBUSTER

Myth: The best time to work out is early in the morning.
Fact: It doesn't matter when you work out, as long as you do so at some point during the day.

THINK DAY 10

Workout: Repeat Range Expander (Think Day 4, page 89)

Goal: Boost flexibility and range of motion

NUTRITION TIP #10

Have a cheat snack every now and then. I like Oreos, personally.

MENTAL CLEANSE #10

Spend some quality time with your family. I don't mean watching TV; I mean talking about events in your community, going for a family hike, or reading a book together.

MYTHBUSTER

Myth: I can turn my muscles into fat if I exercise with weights.

Fact: Fat and muscle are completely different tissues, so you can't transform one into the other. Although muscles can't physically turn into fat, they can atrophy. When you exercise, your initial goal should be to burn fat and build muscle.

PHASE TWO: REACH

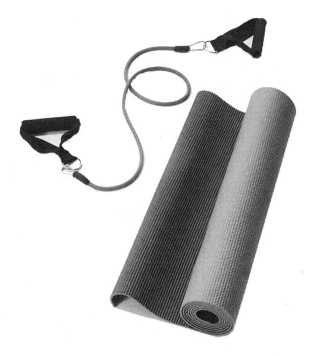

Now that we've built a stable platform of smart nutrition and muscular flexibility, it's time to reach for endurance and power. Aerobic exercises are great for the heart and lungs, but they don't necessarily help your muscles. Both men and women need resistance training to build strong, lean muscles. Because muscles have so much mass, they burn large numbers of calories when they work hard. Resistance training also assists in increasing bone density. That's especially good news for women, who have higher rates of osteoporosis.

In this phase of the program you'll learn how to overcome the resistance of your own body weight, resistance bands, conventional weights, and common household items like cans and chairs. Resistance training is designed to build muscle mass and power. In fitness, power means the ability to move a specific weight load at a specific speed. In life, power means the ability to make someone do something that they wouldn't do on their own. In both fitness and life, you always have two options when you encounter resistance: You can either quit or figure out a way to overcome the resistance. The more you work to overcome resistance, the more power you develop. And the more power you have, the more resistance you can overcome.

REACH DAY 1

NUTRITION TIP #11

Do your nervous system a favor by cutting back on caffeine. Try a cup of herbal tea instead of caffeinated coffee or tea. Herbal tea is soothing to your soul. I drink chamomile tea when I want to relax and ginger tea when I need a little energy boost.

MENTAL CLEANSE #11

Buy a sketch pad and draw something. I don't care if it's a stick figure; just grab your pencil and draw. As you draw, your mind will open up and float free.

Workout: Butt Blaster

Goal: Tighten your butt and your outer and inner thighs

I've yet to meet a client who didn't want to look better in jeans. This workout will get you there!

Note: Start all exercises in standing position, feet shoulder width apart.

SIDE-STEP JACKS

Start with your hands by your sides. Raise your arms out to the sides like you're waving for help. At the same time, step your left leg out to the side while shifting all your weight to your right leg. Bring your arms back down and your legs together. Repeat on the right. Do as many reps as you can in 60 seconds.

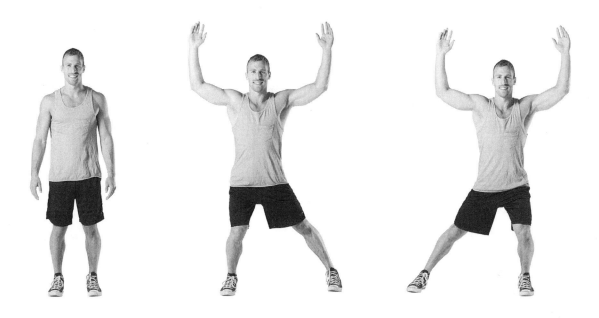

THIGH-BLASTING KICKS

Bring your hands up in fighting position with your fists clenched on either side of your jaw. Keep your abdominals tight and your back straight. Raise your left leg with a bent knee and quickly extend your leg out in front, leaving a very small bend in the knee while punching straight out with your right hand. Return to the starting position and repeat on the right. Go as fast as you can for 60 seconds.

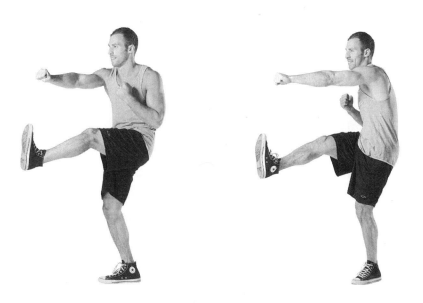

LATERAL SIDE STEP

Place both hands in front of your face as if you were going to catch a ball. Shift all your weight to your left leg. As your weight shifts, move your right leg and then your left leg over to the left in a rapid skipping motion, so that your right foot ends up where your left foot started. Repeat the exercise in the opposite direction, and continue skipping from side to side for 60 seconds.

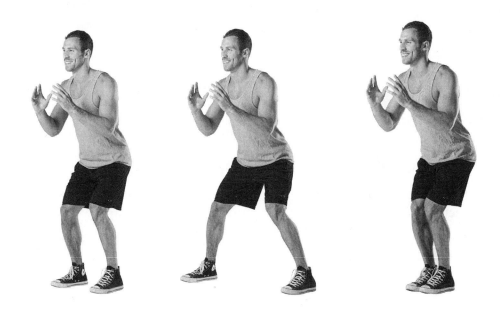

DANCE HALL HOT STEPPER

Pretend you are in a club in Jamaica, rocking to the beat of the drums. Stand with your feet shoulder width apart, knees slightly bent. Step backward with your left leg, touching the floor behind you with the ball of your foot. As your left leg moves backward, swing your left shoulder forward and rotate your torso slightly to the right. Then swing your right shoulder forward, and immediately step forward with your left leg past neutral position, placing your leg in front you and touching the ball of your foot to the floor. Return to neutral position (feet parallel) and then repeat the same steps on the right side. Continue for 60 seconds, alternating sides as fast as you can.

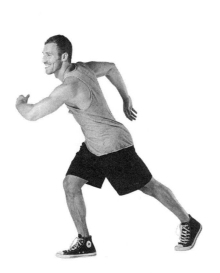

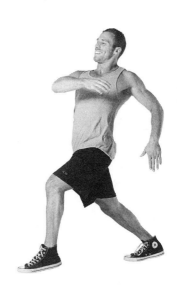

KARATE KID STORK STANCE (LEFT/RIGHT)

Extend both arms horizontally to the sides, parallel to the floor. Flex both wrists downward and squeeze your fingers together the way you would if you were mimicking someone who talks too much. Shift all your weight to your right leg. Raise your left leg with a bent knee as high as you can, and hold it there for 60 seconds. Be sure to keep your abdominals drawn in as tight as possible. Repeat on the right side for another 60 seconds.

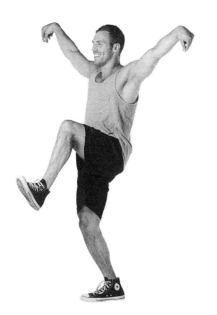

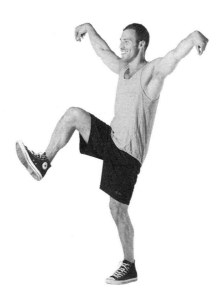

REVERSE LUNGE

Keep your back straight and your abdominals tight. Shift all your weight to your right side. Extend your left leg behind you until your right leg is bent at 90 degrees, keeping the right knee behind the toes. Keep your left leg fully extended with a slight bend at the knee. Simultaneously, touch the floor with your left hand. Repeat for 60 seconds, alternating sides.

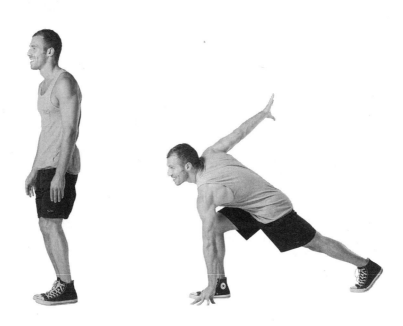

STANDING HYDRANTS (LEFT/RIGHT)

Just like it sounds, this exercise mimics a dog peeing on a hydrant. Stand with your feet together and your knees bent, pushing your butt back and keeping your knees behind your toes. Keeping your chest at a 45-degree angle to the floor, shift all your weight to your right leg. Raise your left heel toward your butt, bending your knee as close to 90 degrees as possible. Next, lift your left leg to the outside of your body so that your inner thigh is parallel to the floor. Return to the original position without touching the floor with your foot. Continue to mark your territory for 60 seconds, then switch sides and repeat for another 60 seconds.

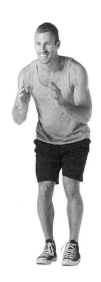 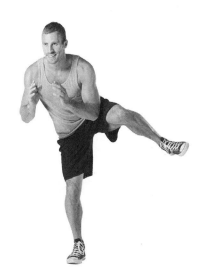

PLIÉ SQUAT

Move your feet a little wider than shoulder width apart, toes pointed outward. Keep a straight back with your arms hanging naturally at your sides. Lower your body by bending your knees while keeping your back straight. Simultaneously, raise both arms like you're about to give me a hug. Squeeze your chest muscles as you bring your hands together. Return to the starting position and repeat for 60 seconds.

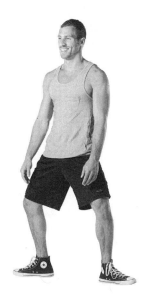 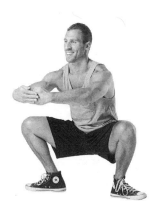

REACH DAY 2

MYTHBUSTER

Myth: Weight lifting is only for men.
Fact: Weight lifting is a great way for both genders to burn calories. Women can benefit particularly from weight training because it increases bone density, which helps you avoid osteoporosis. Also, ladies, targeted weight lifting will help firm and tighten your backside.

Workout: Arm Yourself

Goal: Increase upper-body strength

This workout will increase strength in your arms, chest, and back while burning away the fat on the backs of your arms. You can say good-bye to those bat wings and hello to some great-looking arms.

Note: To avoid injuring your knees, please do these exercises on a carpet or floor mat.

DOLPHIN PUSH-UPS

Lie facedown (prone) with your palms pressed to the floor, parallel to your chest. Keep your elbows tight to your body and your ankles flexed so the balls of your feet touch the floor. Pushing from your palms, lift your chest a few inches off the ground so that you feel tension in your triceps (back of upper arm), but not in your lower back. Return to the starting position and repeat for 30 seconds. Rest for 15 seconds and transition into Modified Push-ups.

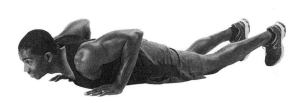
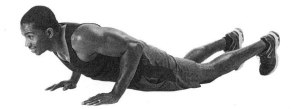

MODIFIED PUSH-UPS

Start as you did for Dolphin Push-ups, except now lift your thighs and chest off the floor while you keep your knees planted. Repeat as fast as you can for 30 seconds. Rest for 15 seconds and then flow into the next exercise, Straight-Arm Plank.

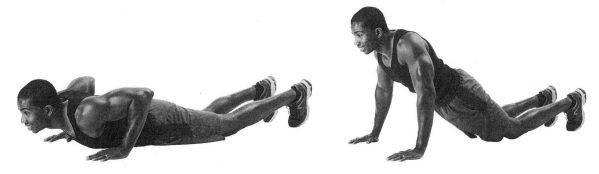

STRAIGHT-ARM PLANK

From the top of the Modified Push-up position, tighten up your butt (gluteus maximus), chest, and abdominals. Next, raise your knees off the ground so your body forms a straight line, parallel to the floor. (**Note:** Make sure there's no curvature in your lower spine.) Hold this position for 30 seconds. Rest for 15 seconds and continue with the next exercise, Walking the Plank.

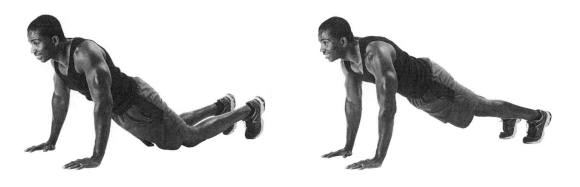

WALKING THE PLANK

Start as you did for Straight-Arm Plank, except keep your knees touching the ground and your elbows bent at 90 degrees and positioned directly below your shoulders, so that your forearms are supporting your body. Shift your weight to the right side and move your left elbow and leg a few inches to the left. Now shift your weight to the left side and move your right elbow and leg to the left, so that you're back in the starting position. Repeat in the opposite direction and continue for 30 seconds, alternating sides.

Note: If this exercise is too easy, try it in full plank position with your knees off the ground (shown here) so that your body forms a straight line.

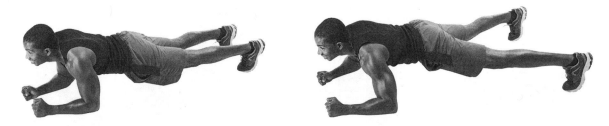

LATE FOR WORK

Pretend you slept through the alarm and now you're late for work. Time to get up! Lie flat on your back (supine), with your legs stretched out. Extend both arms behind your head and melt your lower back into the floor. Swing your arms up and forward, lifting your torso off the ground. Try to touch your toes; then return to the starting position and repeat as fast as you can for 30 seconds.

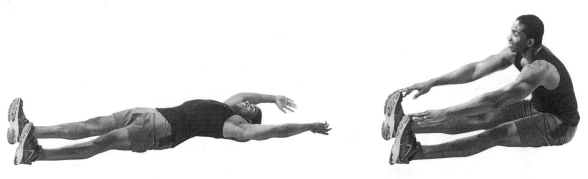

REACH DAY 3

NUTRITION TIP #13

Eat until you feel satisfied, but not full. It takes 30 minutes for your body to digest food, which means that you'll start feeling full half an hour after you eat.

MENTAL CLEANSE #13

Take a shower, get dressed up, and take yourself out somewhere nice like the movies or a play. You've earned it!

MYTHBUSTER

Myth: Lifting weights will make me bulky.

Fact: Weight training accounts for 70 percent of your calorie burn. Resistance forces your muscles to work 10 to 20 times more than regular cardio, without bulking. Bulk comes from high calorie intake, which is why professional bodybuilders consume a lot of calories while lifting a lot of weight. If you combine weight training with a moderate, balanced diet with medium to low calorie intake, you will burn fat and sculpt your body without adding bulk.

Workout: Rubber Soul

Goal: Build upper-body strength

To help build and tone your muscles, we're going to add some external resistance to your workout. We'll start with resistance bands, which are a great alternative to weight training. Compared to weights, bands are kinder on the joints and a whole lot easier to carry in your bag.

Note: This is not a speed workout. I want you to perform each movement as slowly as you can while contracting the muscle that's being worked. The less speed, the more benefit!

STANDING ROW

Stand with your feet shoulder width apart. Wrap the band twice around your knuckles on both sides and make two fists. Extend your arms in front of you, palms down, elbows out and slightly bent. Next, stretch out the band by pulling your elbows behind your body and squeezing your shoulder blades together. Return slowly to the starting position and repeat for 60 seconds.

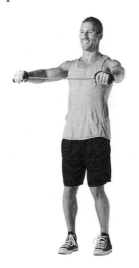
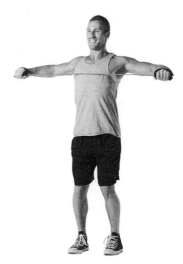

LAT PULL

Start with your arms extended at 45 degrees, fists above your head, elbows slightly bent. Stretch the band out as far as you can by pulling your arms out to the sides until the band just touches the top of your chest. As you stretch the band, push your chest forward slightly and squeeze your shoulder blades together. Return slowly to the starting position and repeat for 60 seconds.

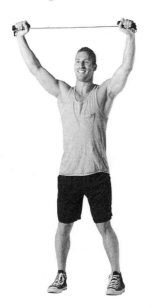
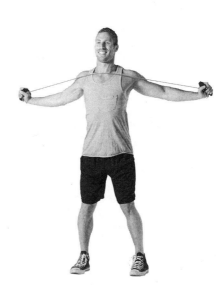

BICEPS CURLS

Stand with your feet shoulder width apart. Holding both handles of the resistance band at your sides, step on the band with both feet. Make sure the band passes under the middle of your feet rather than your toes, to avoid having it snap up and hit you in the face. Keeping your elbows locked to your sides, bend your elbows, bringing your fists up to your chest while squeezing your biceps. Return slowly to the starting position and repeat for 60 seconds.

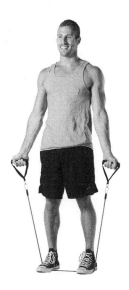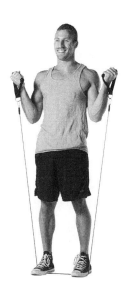

REVERSE FLY

Begin with the starting position you used for the Biceps Curls, except tilt your chest forward at a 45-degree angle. Stretch the band by lifting both elbows to the rear of your body, squeezing your shoulder blades together and tracing the line of your thighs with your hands. When your hands reach your hips, stop and return slowly to the starting position. Repeat for 60 seconds.

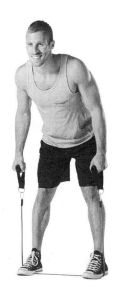 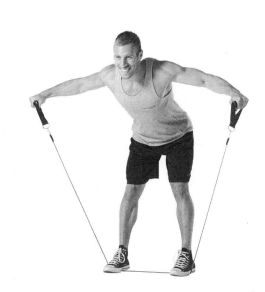

ALTERNATING CURLS

Begin with the starting position you used for the Biceps Curls and continue to use the Biceps Curls movements, but alternate your arms. This isolates each arm and allows you to feel your weak points. Repeat for 60 seconds. Three more sets of the entire workout, and you're done!

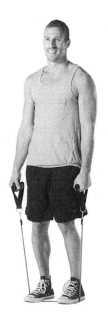 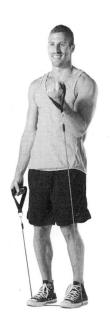 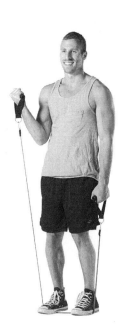

REACH DAY 4

Workout: Yoga Flow

Goal: Increase general flexibility and strength

The human body is not designed to be stiff. You were made to move freely. This workout is based on yoga principles and is designed to build a balance of strength and flexibility. I want you to flow through this routine without pausing between exercises. Don't forget to breathe!

Note: Hold each pose for 30 seconds and then transition right into the next pose. Repeat for a total of 3 rounds.

MOUNTAIN POSE

Stand with your feet together and your hands placed down to the sides with your feet firmly planted on your mat. Pull your abdominals inward, lifting your chest like you're proud of yourself, which you should be! Raise your hands above your head, attempting to bring your hands together.

Note: Press your elbows toward your midline. Try to keep your shoulders from lifting.

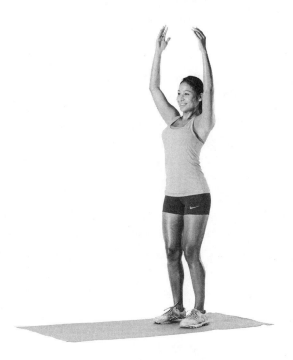

FORWARD BEND

Lower your arms back down to your sides, keeping your feet together and planted firmly. Take a deep breath in and slowly bring your arms down to the floor, bending from your hips. Bring your torso down as far as possible, like you're trying to rest your head on your shins. Keep your knees slightly bent throughout this movement.

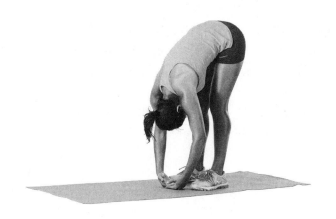

RUNNER'S LUNGE (LEFT)

Extend your left foot backward, keeping it as straight as possible. Keep your right knee bent at a full 90-degree angle. Your right knee should be behind your toes and aligned with your ankle. Your chest should be lifted, keeping your back in a straight line, with no curve whatsoever. Look straight ahead, keeping your spine neutral, and place your hands to the left of your right foot, planted on the floor.

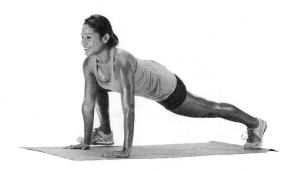

WARRIOR POSE

Lift your torso upright by pressing through the mat with your right heel. Keep your legs in the same position. Your left foot should be turned outward, aligning the left heel with the right heel. Extend your arms out, keeping your palms facing down. I want you to visually try to reach your arms to touch something in the distance both in front of you and behind you. You should feel a deep stretch in both arms. Look straight ahead, keeping your chin parallel to the floor.

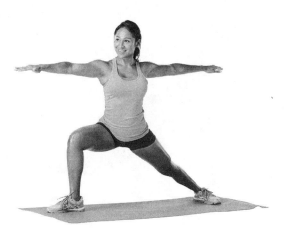

PLANK

Press your palms firmly into your mat, keeping your abdominals tight and your arms fully straight. Your shoulders should be directly over your hands. Step your right leg backward, keeping your body in one straight line parallel to the floor and your eyes looking straight ahead.

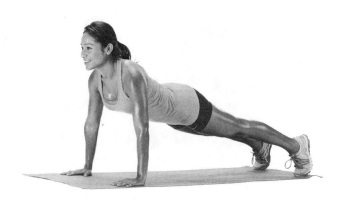

RUNNER'S LUNGE (RIGHT)

Return to the Runner's Lunge pose, this time extending your right leg backward.

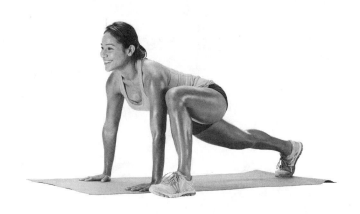

WARRIOR POSE (REDUX)

Lift your torso upright by pressing through the mat with your left heel. Your right foot should be turned outward, aligning the right heel with the left heel. Extend your arms out, keeping your palms facing down. Once again, try to reach your arms to touch something in the distance both in front of you and behind you. You should feel a deep stretch in both arms. Look straight ahead, keeping your chin parallel to the floor.

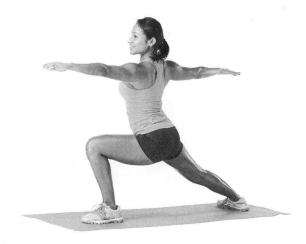

PLANK (REDUX)

Step your left leg backward keeping your body in one straight line parallel to the floor. Press your palms firmly into your mat, keeping your abdominals tight and your arms fully straight. Your shoulders should be directly over your hands.

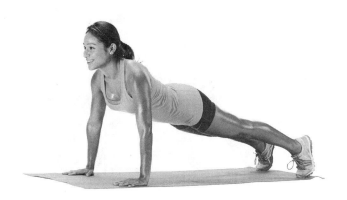

UPWARD DOG

Slowly lower your body down to the floor, keeping your elbows tight to your ribs. Next, press your palms into your mat, breathe out, and push your torso up and away from the floor by extending your elbows until your arms are fully straight. Keep your shoulders relaxed by dropping them down toward the floor. Gaze upward, pointing your chin toward the sky.

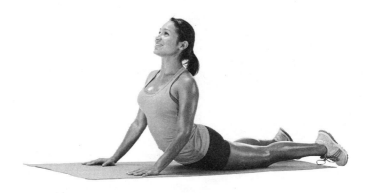

DOWNWARD DOG

From Upward Dog, I want you to push your palms into the mat, raising your hips as high as you can toward the sky. Your hands should be aligned with your hips. Now drop your head, allowing your spine to lengthen. Keep your legs straight and press your heels into the floor. At this point your body should look like an upside-down V.

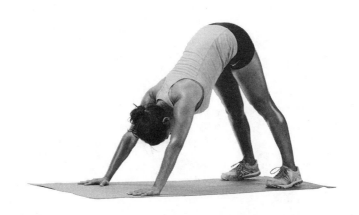

RUNNER'S LUNGE (LEFT)

Return to Runner's Lunge, extending your left leg backward.

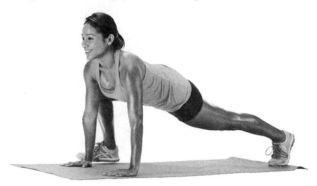

FORWARD BEND

Starting from Runner's Lunge, slowly bring your right foot back next to your left foot. Lift your hips by extending your knees until your legs are nearly straight. Keep your torso bent from the hips and your head still pointed to your shins. Keep your arms extended, with your hands contacting the floor.

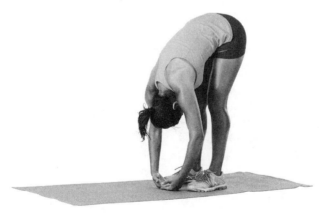

MOUNTAIN POSE

Return to upright position, lifting your torso one vertebra at a time. Extend your arms above your head without raising your shoulders. Your palms should be facing each other and connected if possible.

Note: Remember to press your elbows toward the midline of your body. Repeat the entire sequence once more.

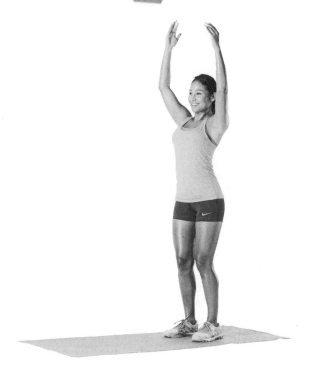

REACH DAY 5

NUTRITION TIP #15

In supermarkets, try to stay in the outside aisles as much as you can. The middle aisles are typically where most of the junk food is. The criminal masterminds who run U.S. supermarkets want you to buy unhealthy processed foods because they are more profitable (for them, not you). That's why they make you walk farther to reach the fruits and vegetables.

MENTAL CLEANSE #15

Learn a new word each day, starting *right now*. Building your vocabulary will increase your brainpower. A person who feels smart can accomplish anything.

Workout: Move Your Butt!

Goal: Strengthen core and lower back

These exercises use resistance from bands and your own body weight.

BAND SQUAT

Stand on your band with your feet slightly wider than your shoulders. Grasp the handles and stretch out the band so that it passes behind your biceps. Push your butt back as you bend your knees, lowering your body as though sinking into a chair. Your knees should now be bent at 90 degrees. Your thighs and butt should be parallel to the floor. Keep your knees behind your toes! Now press through your heels as you stand back up to the starting position. As you return to standing position, tighten your abs and butt by pushing your hips forward.

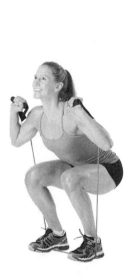
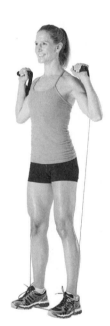

THIGH BLASTER (LEFT AND RIGHT)

Stand on your band with your feet shoulder width apart. Use your right hand to grab the left handle and your left hand to grab the right handle, making an X shape across your thighs with the band. Pull the handles up to your waist and press them firmly against your body. Bend your knees, tighten your abs, and keep your back straight. Now shift all of your weight to your right leg. Soften your knees and kick your left leg out to the side as high as you can. Slowly return your left leg to the starting position. Complete as many reps as possible for a total of 60 seconds, and then repeat on the right side.

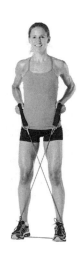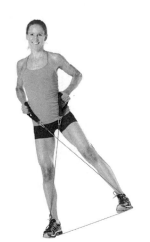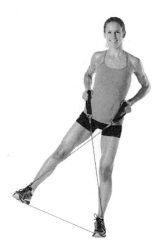

BRIDGE IT UP

Lie on your back and melt your lower back into the floor. Bend your knees and bring your heels as close to your butt as possible. Lift your butt off the floor, raising your hips toward the ceiling as you press your heels into the floor. You should feel a great stretch on the tops of your thighs (quadriceps). Pull your stomach in as tight as you can and clench your butt muscles together. Now your body should look like a perfect bridge. Slowly lower your hips to the floor. Repeat for a total of 60 seconds.

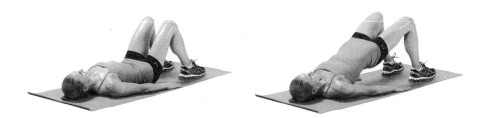

BUTT ENHANCER

Lie facedown on the floor with your arms extended out in front of you. Bend your elbows at 90 degrees, placing your left forearm over your right forearm with your hands touching your elbows. Allow your forehead to rest on your left forearm. Tighten your core and lift your thighs and feet off the ground, using your glutes (butt muscles) and not your lower back. Squeeze your butt as tight as you can and hold for 2 seconds, keeping your toes flexed. Slowly lower your thighs and feet back to the starting position and repeat for a total of 60 seconds.

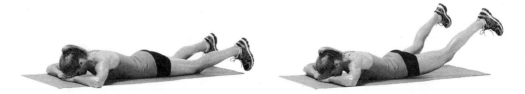

Complete this entire sequence three more times and you're done! Drink some water and then blend up one of my special juice recipes, starting on page 162. You've earned it.

REACH DAY 6

REST DAY!

Go for a bike ride or a relaxing swim, or try one of the Sneak-Attack Workouts starting on page 199.

NUTRITION TIP #16

Chew each bite of food s-l-o-w-l-y. You'll enjoy it more, and your digestive system will thank you.

MENTAL CLEANSE #16

Treat yourself to a social night out with close friends.

MYTHBUSTER

Myth: Exercise is only for adults.
Fact: One in three children in the United States is overweight or obese, according to the American Heart Association. You should certainly encourage your kids to work out and play sports, with the caveat that children under age 12 should avoid exercises that put excessive strain on their developing joints.

REACH DAY 7

I hope you enjoyed your rest day. Now it's time to go hard!

Workout: Repeat Butt Blaster (Reach Day 1, page 104)

Goal: Tighten your butt and your outer and inner thighs

NUTRITION TIP #17

Avoid packaged foods that contain more than 6 ingredients. Donovan's Theorem: More ingredients equal more processing, which equals fewer nutrients.

MENTAL CLEANSE #17

Do a puzzle, aka resistance for your brain. Pick your favorite—jigsaw, Rubik's Cube, math puzzle, whatever it is. Personally, I like crossword puzzles.

MYTHBUSTER

Myth: If I eat more protein I can build big muscles.
Fact: Building muscle mass requires (A) eating more calories than you burn and (B) using enough weight to challenge muscles beyond their normal levels of resistance. You should eat a balanced, healthy diet that includes protein, fat, carbohydrates, fiber, vitamins, and minerals.

REACH DAY 8

Workout: Repeat Rubber Soul (Reach Day 3, page 113)

Goal: Build upper-body strength

NUTRITION TIP #18

Avoid high-fructose corn syrup (HFCS), a common ingredient in most processed foods, including many that claim to be "natural." HFCS activates a hormone in your body called ghrelin, which makes you feel hungry more often.

MENTAL CLEANSE #18

The news is full of negativity, which will drag you down. Turn it off and spend 5 minutes listening to whatever kind of music you find most relaxing. For me it's cultural reggae, like Bob Marley or Morgan Heritage.

REACH DAY 9

Workout: Repeat Yoga Flow (Reach Day 4, page 117)

Goal: Increase general flexibility and strength

NUTRITION TIP #19

Avoid eating at open buffets, which are like happy hour for harmful bacteria. Instead, pack a cooler with healthy homemade food (see page 49).

MENTAL CLEANSE #19

Now that you've started breaking those old habits that were dragging you down, it's time to try something new. Today try a new route to work or a new recipe. (I have some great ones for you to try, starting on page 157.)

REACH DAY 10

Workout: Repeat Move Your Butt! (Reach Day 5, page 124)

Goal: Strengthen core and lower back

NUTRITION TIP #20

Drink when you are thirsty. This will help your body flush out toxins and transport nutrients to your cells.

MENTAL CLEANSE #20

Refrain from the use of any foul language today. Keep your mouth clean and let only positive words come out of it. You owe that to yourself.

PHASE THREE: MOVE

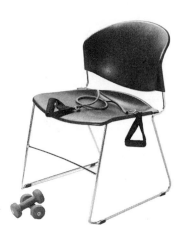

At this point in the No Excuses program, it's time to pick up the pace. Move exercises are based on my original synthesis of martial arts and circuit training, where you move from exercise to exercise with little or no rest in between. It's all about speed, which you can't achieve without flexibility, endurance, and power.

In a typical Move sequence, you execute a series of hard-core defensive movements, such as fist strikes, front kicks, and outside crescent kicks. You intersperse the defensive moves with speed-driven abdominal crunches, squat thrusts, and push-ups. The pace is fast because the goal is to bring your heart rate up and push your body to the point of muscular failure. Let's move!

MOVE DAY 1

NUTRITION TIP #21

Cut back on dairy products, which are loaded with sugar and saturated fats. Try substituting almond, soy, or coconut milk.

MENTAL CLEANSE #21

Now that you've come this far in the program, it's time to start giving back. Today I want you to volunteer your services to help others meet their challenges. One of my favorite things to do is help kids understand more about fitness.

Workout: Just for Kicks

Goal: Build strength, speed, power, and balance

Kicking is one of the foundations of the martial arts. It strengthens your core, improves overall body strength, and burns a ton of calories. So let's start kicking!

FRONT STRETCH KICK (LEFT AND RIGHT)

Stand with your right foot forward and your left foot back. Bend your arms and bring your fists toward the sides of your cheeks as if you were getting ready to brawl. Soften your knees. Now shift all your weight to your right leg and kick forward with your left leg as high as you can, keeping your kicking leg straight with your toes pointed up to the ceiling. Do as many kicks as you can in 30 seconds, then switch legs and kick for another 30 seconds.

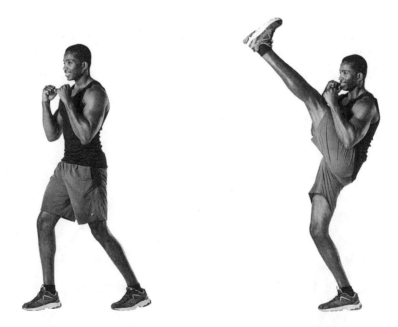

SIDE STRETCH KICK (LEFT AND RIGHT)

Stand with your feet shoulder width apart. Bring your hands up in fighting position, and soften your knees. Kick your left leg out to the side, extending it fully while pointing your toes up to the ceiling. Do as many kicks as you can in 30 seconds, then switch legs and kick for another 30 seconds.

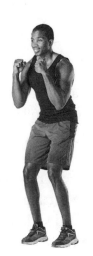
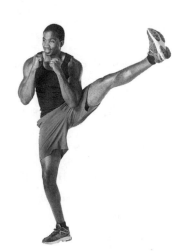

SWING KICK (LEFT AND RIGHT)

Begin with the same stance you took in Side Stretch Kick. Kick your left leg forward, then swing it back behind you and return to the starting position. Your foot should not touch the ground during this kick. Do as many kicks as you can in 30 seconds, then switch legs and kick for another 30 seconds.

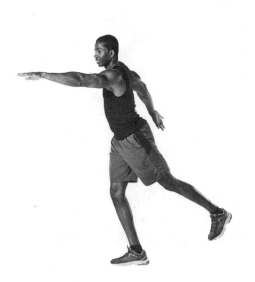
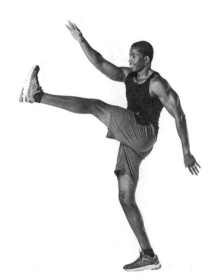

OUTSIDE CRESCENT KICK (LEFT AND RIGHT)

Stand with your right foot forward and your left foot back. Kick with your left leg to the far right side, carry your left leg back across your body to the far left side, then return to the starting position. Do as many kicks as you can in 30 seconds, then switch legs and kick for another 30 seconds.

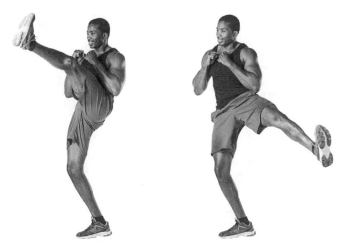

INSIDE CRESCENT KICK

Begin in the same starting position you took for the Outside Crescent Kick, and use the same moves, but backward: Swing your back leg out and across to the opposite side, then pull it back across your body to the starting position. Do as many kicks as you can in 30 seconds, then switch legs and kick for another 30 seconds.

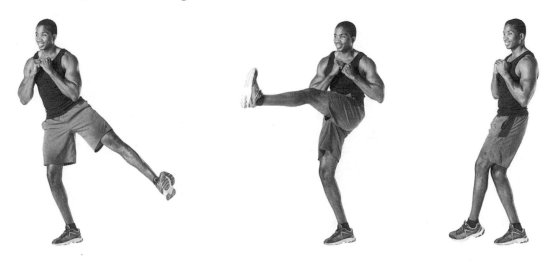

ALTERNATING KNEES

Stand with your feet parallel and shoulder width part, your knees soft, and your hands in fighting position. Bring your left leg up as high as you can, toes pointing to the floor. Repeat for 60 seconds, alternating knees.

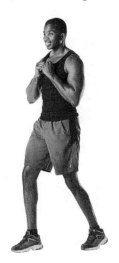
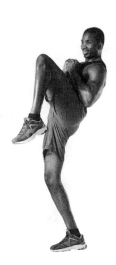

SQUAT TO KNEE

Stand with your feet parallel, slightly wider than your shoulders, hands in fighting stance. Pretend you're sitting down in a chair, pushing your butt backward. Rise back to the starting position, pushing through your heels, and simultaneously lift your left knee as high as you can. Repeat for 60 seconds, alternating knee lifts.

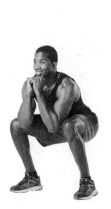
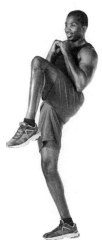

SINGLE LEG KICK ON ONE LEG

Stand with your right foot forward and your left foot back. Move your rear leg forward, lifting your knee, then extend your leg in a kick, keeping your toes pointed forward. Repeat for 30 seconds, then switch to your right leg and kick for another 30 seconds.

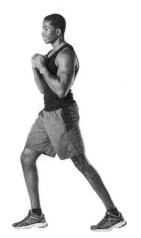 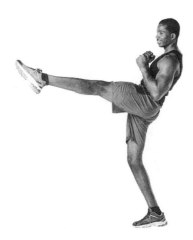

SIDE KICK

Stand with your feet parallel, in a wide stance, hands in fighting position. Rotate your right foot so your toes are pointed away from your body, perpendicular to your left foot. Shift your left foot so your heel is pointing to the left side of your body. Place all your weight on your right leg, lifting your left leg as high as you can, pulling your toes in. Extend your left leg out, pointing your heel toward the target. Look left, pick a target, and stay focused on it. Repeat for 30 seconds, then switch to the right side.

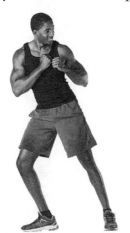 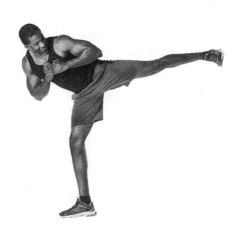

PUSH KICK

Stand with your right foot forward and your left foot back. Lift your rear leg forward and up as high as you can, bending the knee. Close your torso over the raised knee. Pop your chest out, pull your elbows back, and thrust your hips forward while extending your leg, keeping your toes pointed to the ceiling. Visualize yourself kicking in a door like some badass ninja. Repeat with the other leg for 60 seconds.

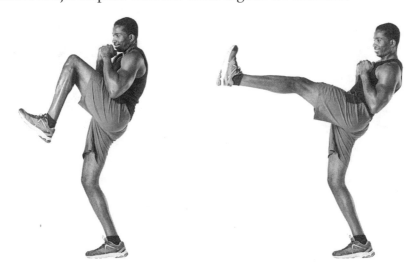

Repeat the entire sequence once. You're done!

MOVE DAY 2

NUTRITION TIP #22

Cut your risk of heart disease by eliminating trans fats from your diet. Trans fats are oils produced by an artificial process called hydrogenation. Fried food is particularly high in trans fats and saturated fats, both of which will grease your path to coronary heart disease.

MENTAL CLEANSE #22

Turn off your phone, put away your damn iPad, and read a real book, made out of paper with words printed on it. It takes strength to do this, but if you've come this far in the program, you can handle it. Choose a book that inspires you to achieve your goals. One of my favorite books is *The Power of Focus*, by Jack Canfield, Mark Victor Hansen, and Les Hewitt. It helped me get to know myself.

Workout: Lose That Thut

Goal: Tighten and strengthen your thighs and gluteus maximus (aka your butt)

I designed this workout especially for those whose butt and thighs have merged into a single, shapeless "thut." This workout will literally get your butt in gear. Bonus: By losing the thut, you'll strengthen the muscles of your lower back, reducing the risk of back injury. Additional bonus: You'll look great in a swimsuit!

BUTT ENHANCER

Lie facedown on the floor with your palms facing down and your arms bent at 90 degrees, like you're one of the cowering customers during a bank robbery. Pull your elbows down toward your ribs, tighten your core, and lift your thighs and feet off the ground, using your glutes (butt) and not your lower back. Squeeze your butt as tight as you can, and hold. Extend your arms straight out in front of you while simultaneously separating your legs, keeping your thighs parallel to the floor. Slowly return your arms and legs to the starting position and repeat for a total of 60 seconds.

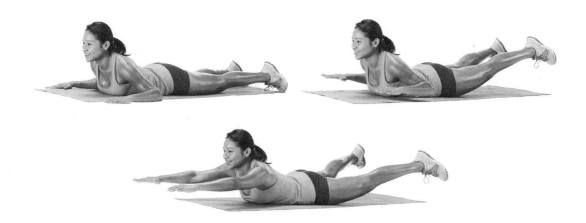

KNEELING HYDRANT WITH BACK KICK (LEFT/RIGHT)

Start on your hands and knees, maintaining a straight back. Shift all of your weight to your right knee and lift your left leg out to the side as high as possible, keeping your knees bent at 90 degrees and your abs tight. Return your left leg toward the midline of your body and then kick the same leg straight back behind, keeping your glutes tight. Return to the starting position and repeat for 60 seconds on each side.

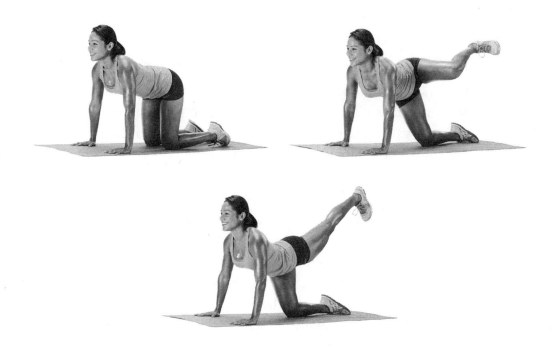

WALKING MOUNTAIN CLIMBERS (LEFT/RIGHT)

Place your body in push-up position with your arms extended, elbows slightly bent, and palms pressed into the ground. Center your body weight, tighten your core, and move your left knee up toward the outside of your left elbow. Plant your left foot on the floor. Keep your right leg straight behind you with a slight bend in the knee. Return the left leg back to the starting position and alternate to the right side. Repeat for 60 seconds as if you were climbing a hill.

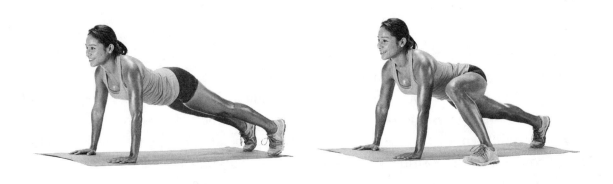

GET YOUR BUTT IN GEAR (LEFT/RIGHT)

Start on all fours, eyes forward. Extend your left leg straight out behind you, keeping your thigh high enough to feel tightness in your left butt cheek. Your toes should be flexed toward your shin. Next, bend your knee to 90 degrees by pulling your left heel toward your butt and flexing the back of your thigh. Slowly kick your left heel up to the ceiling, keeping your toes flexed toward your shin and your butt tight. Repeat for 60 seconds on each side.

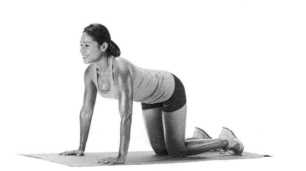 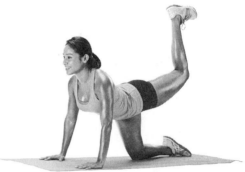

Repeat the entire sequence four more times and you are done!

MOVE DAY 3

Workout: Jump Street

Goal: Build overall strength and range of motion

I designed this workout to boost speed and power in your legs and shoulders. You'll learn how to move your shoulders through a broad range of motions, which most people don't know how to do. This workout will also develop your jumping ability, which is helpful if you need to jump out of (or into) a window, over a car, or simply out of the way.

STANDING FRONT AND SIDE RAISE

Step on your resistance band with your feet shoulder width apart, holding the handles next to your hips. Lift your chest and tighten your abdominals as you lift your arms until they are fully extended and parallel to the floor. Now squeeze your chest together as you bring your hands together in front of your chest. Keep your palms facing down. Move your arms back to the raised side position and then lower them back down to your hips. Complete as many rounds as you can for a total of 60 seconds.

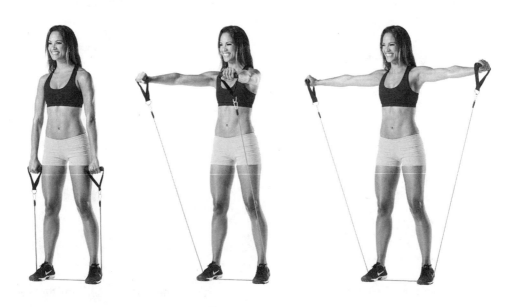

MIKE TYSON KNOCKOUT PUNCH

Step on your band with your feet a little wider than shoulder width apart. Bend your knees and firmly grasp the handles with tight fists facing outward. Bend your elbows to 90 degrees, bringing your fists up to your torso. Punch the sky with your left arm while keeping your right arm still. As you lower your left arm, punch upward with your right arm. Go for the knockout, alternating punches as fast as you can for 60 seconds.

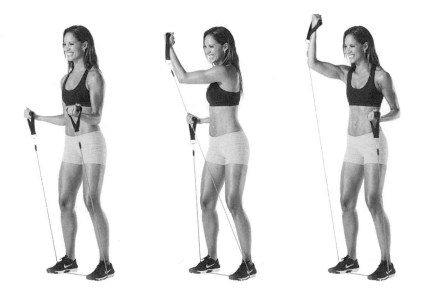

MOVE IT!

You don't need the band for this one. Stand with your feet wider than shoulder width apart. Bend your knees slightly and bring your hands up to your chest as if you were going to catch a ball. Shift your weight to your left leg and quickly skip left, bringing your right foot in the place of your left foot. Squat down and touch the floor with your left hand. Now skip across to the right side, and squat and touch the floor with your right hand. Pretend a truck is barreling toward you at full speed and you have to get your butt out of the way.

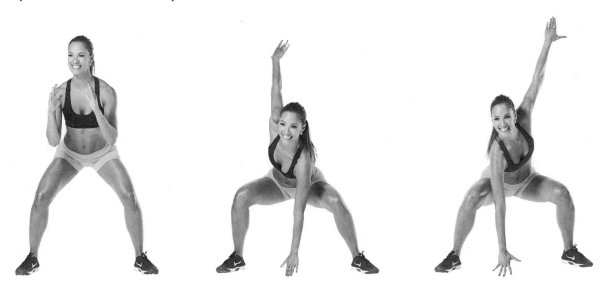

REBOUNDER

Stand with your feet shoulder width apart. Bend your knees at 90 degrees and tilt your chest forward, pulling your arms behind you. Keep your arms straight and tight to your body as if you were getting ready to jump for a rebound in basketball. Now shift to the balls of your feet. Swing your arms up to the ceiling and jump as high as you can, landing back in the starting position. Repeat for a total of 60 seconds.

Note: If you have knee problems, don't jump. Instead simply rise onto the balls of your feet without leaving the ground.

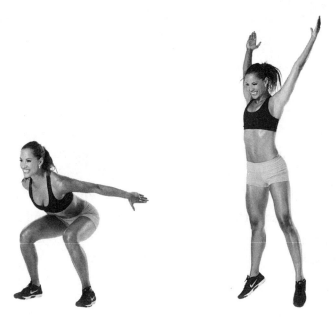

CHEERLEADER

Stand with both your knees bent at 90 degrees, feet shoulder width apart. Cross your arms and lower your hands nearly to the floor, pushing your butt back. Keep your knees behind your toes and your back flat like a tabletop. Now jump as high as you can, extending your arms up and to the sides while spreading your legs apart in the air. Your body should look like a perfect X. Think of yourself as a cheerleader cheering me on for more books to come. *Go, Donovan!* Land softly in the starting position and repeat as fast as you can for 60 seconds.

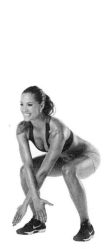
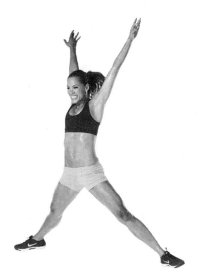

Repeat entire sequence three more times and you are done!

MOVE DAY 4

NUTRITION TIP #24

If you want to lose weight, don't add sweeteners to your food. Much of the food we eat already contains natural sugars.

MENTAL CLEANSE #24

Buy your boss a small treat like a cup of coffee even if he or she is a jerk. And if you are the jerk (boss), do the same for your employees. Making a small human gesture will add some warmth to those relationships and do wonders for your soul.

Workout: Powerhouse Knockout

Goal: Build stamina, strength, and speed

In this workout you'll punch negative thoughts straight out the window using moves from boxing and kickboxing. You will need a light pair of dumbbells, so go get 'em— 2 to 5 pounds is optimal. If you don't have dumbbells, I'll wait until you buy some. Alternatively, grab a couple of cans of soup or beans from the kitchen.

Note: Start all moves with your feet shoulder width apart, knees slightly bent, and abs tight.

SUPER(WO)MAN POWER PUNCH

Grasping your dumbbells firmly, bring your fists up to the sides of your jaw in fighting position. Put on your war face and punch as fast as you can, alternating left and right. Repeat for a total of 60 seconds.

Note: To avoid hyperextending your elbows, end each punch with your elbow slightly bent.

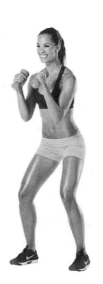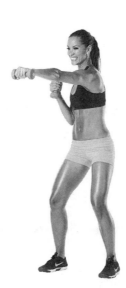

ARE YOU TALKING TO ME? (LEFT/RIGHT)

Hold your dumbbells firmly in both hands. Raise your arms in front of you, elbows bent at 45 degrees. Place your left leg behind you and keep your right leg bent in front of you. Shift all of your weight to your right leg. Aggressively pull your arms down to your torso while you lift your left knee as high as you can. I want you to pretend that you are grabbing someone by the collar and kneeing them in the groin at the same time. Go as fast as you can on your left side for 60 seconds. Repeat on your right side for another 60 seconds.

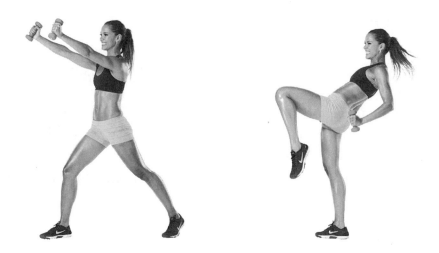

POW, WOW! (LEFT/RIGHT)

In certain social situations, it is perfectly appropriate to elbow your interlocutor in the face and then kick them through the wall. Here's how: Hold the dumbbells on both sides of your jaw, keeping your elbows tight to your sides. Your first move is your elbow strike. Push your left fist across to your right side while protecting your right jaw with the right fist. Next, strike rapidly sideways with your left elbow while keeping your fist facing down to the floor. Return to the starting position. Turn your right foot out and shift all your weight to your right leg. Lift your left leg up with your toes flexed. Turn your left butt cheek in the direction you are kicking, quickly extend your leg, and then return to the starting position. Repeat for 60 seconds on each side.

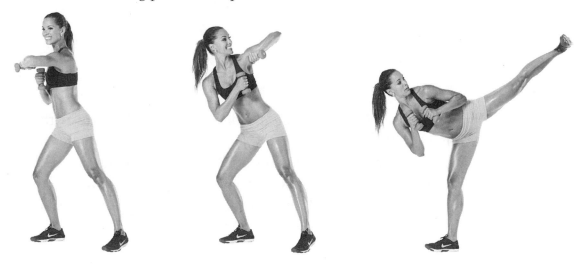

KICK 'EM WHERE IT HURTS

This is the move that wins fights, and I have my money on *you*! Raise your dumbbells with your arms at 90 degrees while squeezing your arm muscles. Shift your weight to your right side and immediately kick your left leg straight out in front of you, pushing your hips forward. Imagine you are kicking an assailant in the groin while aggressively pulling your arms down to your sides and tightening your triceps. Alternate kicks on both sides as fast as you can for 60 seconds.

    Note: Keep your kicking leg slightly bent to avoid hyperextension of the knee.

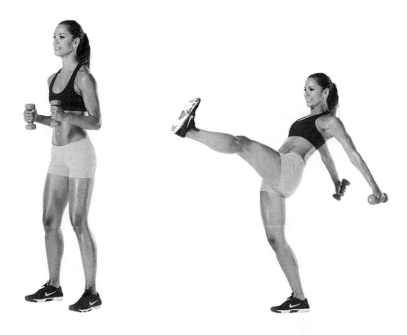

TAP THAT CHIN

Pretend you are ducking away from a punch and then returning the favor with two uppercuts to the chin. Hold the dumbbells in front of your jaw with your palms facing inward. Push your butt back parallel to the floor as if you were sinking into a chair. Keep your knees behind your toes. Press back upright from your heels while punching up to the ceiling, alternating left and right punches. Repeat as fast as possible for 60 seconds.

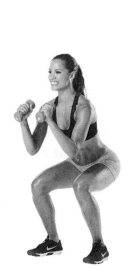
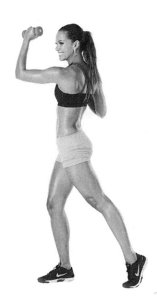

GET OFF ME!

Lie flat on your back with your knees bent, your heels planted into the floor, and both arms at 90 degrees. Tighten your stomach and raise your torso off the ground by curling your spine one vertebrae at a time. Stop at a 45-degree angle or wherever you feel your stomach muscles are really tight. Twist your waist to the right, bringing your right shoulder back and your left shoulder forward. Punch across the body with your left fist and return to the starting position. Next, punch left with your right fist and return to the starting position. Lie back on the floor and repeat for a total of 60 seconds, moving as fast as you can.

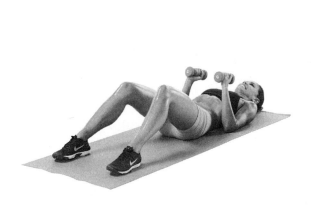
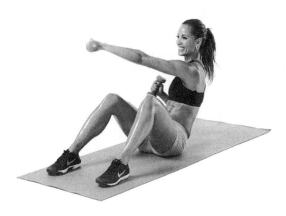

QUICK HANDS SHOULDER TAPS

Assume a position on all fours, hands and knees shoulder width apart. Press your palms into the ground and lift your knees away from the floor, planting the balls of your feet. Your body should now be in plank position, forming a straight line. Tighten your abdominals and your entire lower body (legs, butt, and inner thighs). Shift all your weight to your right arm, keeping your hips parallel to the floor, and quickly touch your right shoulder with your left hand. Immediately repeat on your right side. Continue as fast as you can for 60 seconds.

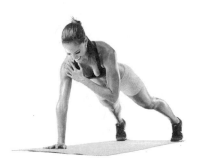 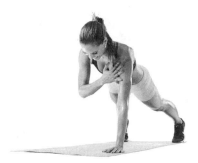

HOLD THAT POSE

Assume a position on all fours, hands and knees shoulder width apart. Bend your elbows, pressing your forearms into the ground. Press your palms together as though praying for world peace. Now lift your knees away from the floor, extending your left leg back, followed by your right leg, and planting the balls of your feet. You are now in elbow plank position. Tighten your abdominals and squeeze your entire lower body. Roll your hips, eliminating the curve in your lower back. Hold the pose for 60 seconds. **Note:** If the full plank position is too difficult, simply keep your knees on the ground.

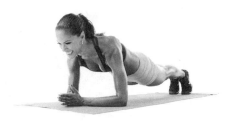

MOVE DAY 5

Workout: HIIT Man (High-Intensity Interval Training)

Goal: General strength and endurance

If you've ever been sedentary, you know that chairs are traps. This workout uses an ordinary kitchen chair (no wheels) as a tool to build strength and stamina. Do each move for 20 seconds with 10 seconds of rest in between moves, for a total of 8 full rounds.

BAT-WING ANNIHILATOR

Sit on the edge of the chair with your palms pressed into the seat. Slide your butt off the chair, keeping your knees bent and using your arms to support your body weight. Keeping your butt close to the chair and your arms close to your sides, lower your torso toward the floor until your elbows reach a 90-degree angle. Press back up to the top until your arms are fully extended. Complete as many reps as you can for 20 seconds. Rest for 10 seconds and continue for another 7 rounds.

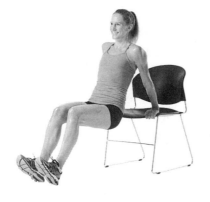 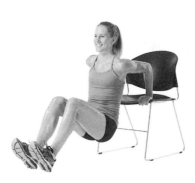

SIDE STEPPER

Stand facing away from your chair. Get down on your hands and knees, palms flat on the floor. Press your palms into the floor with your arms fully extended, using your arms to support your weight. Lift your left leg, followed by your right leg, and place them firmly on your chair seat, so that the balls of your feet are pressing into the chair. Tighten your abs and keep your weight centered. Now you're in plank position, with your body forming a straight line. Clench your left butt cheek and lift your left leg off the chair. Move your leg out to the side and down, touching the floor with your foot. Lift that leg and return it to the seat of the chair. Do the same for your right side. Complete as many reps as you can for 20 seconds. Rest for 10 and go again for another 7 rounds.

Note: If it's too hard to do the exercise with your feet up on the chair, substitute a normal plank position with your feet on the ground.

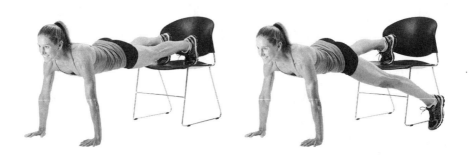

GET UP, GET DOWN

Sit at the edge of the chair, feet at shoulder width and fists next to your jaw in fighting position. Next, press through your heels, bringing your chest forward just enough to stand. Once upright, tighten up your butt. Kick your left and then your right leg out in front of you, keeping your knees soft. Place both feet back together and planted to the floor. Bend at the waist, look backward through your legs, and sit back on the chair. Complete as many reps as you can for 20 seconds. Rest for 10 seconds and go again for another 7 rounds.

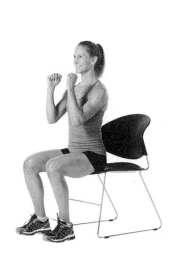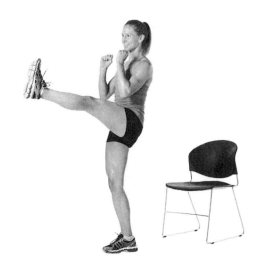

AB BLASTER

Lie on your back with both feet resting on the seat of the chair, soles touching the back-rest. Keep your arms at your sides, palms down. Depending on the height of the chair, your knees should be bent as close as possible to 90 degrees. Next, lift your head off the floor, rolling your upper shoulders off the ground. At the same time, lift your arms to the height of the chair seat. Tighten your abs and curl your body up aggressively, touching the seat with your hands as close to your feet as possible. Your goal is to touch your ankles. Repeat for 20 seconds, rest for 10 seconds, and continue for another 7 rounds.

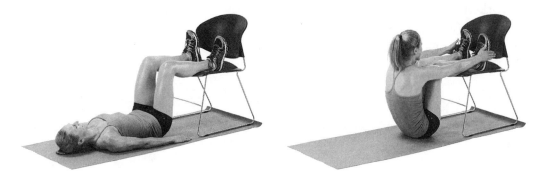

CHAIR SQUAT

Stand with your feet wider than your shoulders. Pick the chair up by grasping both rear legs just under the seat. Extend your arms in front of you with a slight bend to your elbows. Push your butt back and bend your knees to 90 degrees, until your butt is parallel to the floor. Keep your upper body as vertical as possible. Stand up by pressing through your heels, with the chair still extended in front of your chest. Then pull the chair in toward your chest, squeezing your shoulder blades together. Repeat for 20 seconds, rest for 10 seconds, continue for 7 more rounds, and you are done!

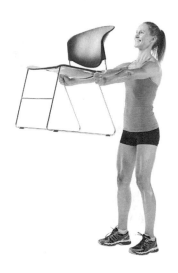
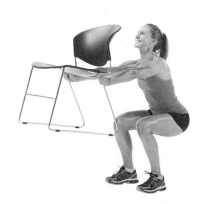

MOVE DAY 6

REST DAY!

You've worked very hard for the past few days. Now it's time to kick back and get loose! Don't slack off on nutrition, but take a break from your regular workout. Instead, work on your flexibility by trying the stretches on page 193.

NUTRITION TIP #26

Fast for a day, consuming only water. Just like your muscles, your intestines need rest time in order to function at their best. If you're not ready for a water fast, try drinking freshly juiced vegetables throughout the day.

Note: It's best to fast on a day when you aren't working out. Try it today!

MENTAL CLEANSE #26

If you've made it this far in the No Excuses program, you should be able to describe yourself in a single word. Find one word that describes your best self. The word that describes me is "elite."

MYTHBUSTER

Myth: I can lose weight by skipping meals.

Fact: This is actually harmful to your body. Skipping meals encourages your body to use protein for energy, which usually means loss of muscle tissue. If you really want to lose weight, you should eat six small healthy meals a day. This will keep your metabolism burning efficiently.

MOVE DAY 7

Workout: Repeat Just for Kicks (Move Day 1, page 131)

Goal: Build strength, speed, power, and balance

NUTRITION TIP #27

Eat more oily fish, such as salmon or mackerel. This is a great way to get more healthy omega-3 fatty acids in your diet. If you don't like fish, substitute a trusted supplement of your choice.

MENTAL CLEANSE #27

Take 5 minutes out of your day to write down all the things that you are thankful for. Try not to think at all about what's wrong with your life. Instead, focus on feeling grateful for what you have. I'm grateful for my amazing family, my health, and my work.

MYTHBUSTER

Myth: You should eliminate certain food groups, such as fat and sugar, from your diet.

Fact: A balanced diet is key to achieving and maintaining weight loss. When you ban entire food groups, you risk creating vitamin deficiencies.

MOVE DAY 8

Workout: Repeat Lose That Thut (Move Day 2, page 137)

Goal: Tighten and strengthen your thighs and gluteus maximus (aka your butt)

NUTRITION TIP #28

Balance your metabolism by consuming a protein, fat, and carbohydrate in each and every meal. The recipes in the back of this book are a great place to start.

MENTAL CLEANSE #28

Call an old friend with whom you have lost touch, maybe over some old grudge. Make peace. It does wonders for the soul.

MYTHBUSTER

Myth: Home workouts are better than going to the gym.

Fact: Some folks find it easier to stick to a home-based fitness program. Others prefer the companionship and sophisticated equipment that you find in a gym. Bottom line: The best workout program is the one you will participate in consistently.

MOVE DAY 9

Workout: Repeat Jump Street (Move Day 3, page 139)

Goal: Build overall strength and range of motion

NUTRITION TIP #29

Keep your refrigerator stocked. (See the pantry list on page 189.) It's easier to make bad food choices if you don't have the right supplies on hand.

MENTAL CLEANSE #29

Think about a specific fear that you have, and find a way to confront it. When my son Dorian was three, he got over his fear of water by simply jumping into the pool. (I was right there by his side, of course.) Now he swims like a fish.

MYTHBUSTER

Myth: Muscle weighs more than fat.

Fact: A pound of muscle and a pound of fat weigh the same, a pound. However, muscles are denser than fat and occupy less space. Adding muscle to your physique will create curves where once there were none.

MOVE DAY 10

Workout: Repeat Powerhouse Knockout (Move Day 4, page 143)

Goal: Build stamina, strength, and speed

NUTRITION TIP #30

Avoid eating heavy foods late at night. Your body will not be able to burn off those calories as you sleep.

MENTAL CLEANSE #30

Make a bucket list. Write down all the things you want to do before you transition from this earth. Think how far you've come in the past 30 days. Now that you've learned to Think, Reach, and Move, how do you want to spend the rest of your life?

MYTHBUSTER

Myth: If I'm not sore the next day, I didn't work out hard enough.

Fact: Soreness is not a reliable indicator of a good workout. It's normal to experience some soreness after a workout, especially if you regularly change your routine. Soreness can also be a sign that you pushed your body too hard. I enjoy feeling sore, but that's just me. The key is to make sure that you're challenging your muscles to their fullest potential.

CONGRATULATIONS!

I'm so proud of you for completing my 30-day No Excuses program. You worked hard, went through hell and back, and showed yourself and the world what you are made of.

A few last words of advice: This is just the beginning of a never-ending battle. In the martial arts I learned that once you earn your black belt you become a white belt all over again. Nobody ever achieves true mastery because we are all students in life. Well, you just earned your black belt. I don't want you to slack off just because you made it past the 30 days. Instead I want you to continue in the program until it becomes embedded in your brain like a computer code.

What you worked so hard to gain can easily be lost. Hold on to it and cherish this achievement. You have made some exciting changes in your life, but there is a whole lifetime of progress ahead of you.

I invite you to join me and a community of like-minded people who are looking to transform their bodies and their lives. Visit me at www.projectslimdown.com and join the movement. Best wishes for continued success.

Peace and blessings,
Donovan Green

CHAPTER 8

RECIPES

One of the main excuses my clients use for not eating right is that they don't have time to cook. I personally love to cook, but I also don't have hours on end to fiddle around in the kitchen. I'm going to give you some of my favorite recipes, all of which are designed to deliver maximum flavor and nutritional benefit with minimum prep time.

Note: Many of these recipes yield more than one serving. You can either share with your family and friends, or store leftovers in the fridge so you always have food ready during the week.

SMOOTHIES

Let's start your nutrition makeover with some of my favorite slim-down smoothies. I have a variety of offerings—sweet and savory, chunky and smooth, thin and thick, sweet and tangy—and endless combinations thereof. Easy to make, refreshing, and satisfying, they will refresh your palate in four quick steps and with a few staple ingredients. A perfect snack for any time of day, they can also serve as a complete meal with some added protein, good fats, or fiber in the form of protein powder and flaxseed.

Making delicious smoothies requires fresh ingredients, a high-capacity blender (at least 1,500 watts), and a couple of minutes of your time to do the following:

1. Place all ingredients in your blender in the order listed.
2. Set your blender on low.
3. Turn on the machine and quickly increase the speed to high.
4. Blend for 30 seconds or until your desired texture and consistency are reached.

Note: Feel free to substitute ingredients, within reason. A mango and a banana are not interchangeable, but if you're craving sweet fruit for your smoothie, don't run out to the store if you have one but not the other. If the recipe calls for agave and you have only honey, use honey. (Natural sweeteners are always preferable to refined sugars because the latter are easier for your body to break down and store as fat.) I don't recommend dairy products, which are high in fat and sugar. Instead, try one of the many natural milk substitutes on the market. I like almond milk, but feel free to substitute coconut, rice, or soy milk if you are allergic to almonds or simply don't like the taste.

Each smoothie recipe yields one to two servings. I recommend that you drink each smoothie right after you make it, when the ingredients are freshest and will deliver the most nutritional value. However, you can store a smoothie in the fridge for an hour or so if you stir in a little lemon juice. This preserves the enzymes in the ingredients and slows the process of oxidization, which causes discoloring. (The same trick works for apple slices.)

Funky Kingston Smoothie

1 cup dry oatmeal (I'd go with rolled oats—steel-cut oats are a bit healthier, but you have to soak them overnight. Avoid instant oatmeal, which has had most of the nutrients processed out of it.)
1 banana
2 tablespoons natural peanut butter (I prefer organic PB, although it is a bit more expensive.)
Dash of ground cinnamon
1 scoop protein powder (Scoop sizes vary—use the one that comes in the jar.)
1 cup unsweetened almond milk
2 tablespoons flaxseed
6 ice cubes

Serves 2

Caribbean Blast

1 cup mango slices
½ cup cantaloupe
1 kiwi, peeled
½ cup ice
½ cup water (more if you prefer the smoothie thinned out)

Serves 2

Protein Power Hit

1 cup unsweetened almond milk
½ cup rolled oats
1 tablespoon natural peanut butter
1 banana
Dash of grated nutmeg
6 ice cubes

Serves 2

Rejuvenator

Handful of blueberries
Handful of raspberries
6 strawberries
½ cup water
3 ice cubes

Serves 1

WHOLE OR SKIM MILK?

I tend to avoid dairy milk altogether because it's high in sugar and fat, and also because I don't like the taste. Skim milk obviously contains less fat than whole milk, but skim is also less satisfying, which can promote overeating. Many nutritionists believe strongly in the health benefits of milk, and there's certainly evidence that dairy helps your body synthesize muscle protein. It also provides good cholesterol, which lowers your risk of stroke and heart attack. I'm not a scientist, so I can only tell you what has worked for my clients and me. If weight loss is a priority for you, I strongly recommend that you cut back on dairy milk. Instead, substitute almond, rice, or soy milk.

Green Monster

Handful of spinach
½ medium cucumber
2 stalks celery
1 green apple, peeled, cored, and quartered
1-inch piece of peeled ginger, grated

1 tablespoon lemon juice
6 ice cubes
1 cup water

Serves 1

Peach Mango Slim Breeze

½ cup water
1 cup mango slices (or flesh of 1 mango)
1 medium peach, pitted and sliced
1 tablespoon raw honey
6 ice cubes

Serves 1

Power Up and Go

1 medium orange, peeled and seeded
1 medium slice canteloupe
1 small green apple, peeled, cored, and quartered
1 banana
6 ice cubes

Serves 1

Watermelon Explosion

2 slices watermelon, cubed
½ large pink grapefruit, coarsely chopped
1 kiwi, peeled
2 tablespoons natural honey
6 ice cubes

Serves 1

Supercharged Lemonade

1 lemon
2 kiwis, peeled
6 ice cubes

Serves 1

Blood Builder

Handful of spinach
½ cup parsley
1 green apple, peeled, cored, and quartered
8 green grapes
4 stalks celery
¼ avocado
⅓ cup water

Serves 1

Slim Slim

1-inch piece of ginger, peeled and grated (use less ginger
    if you want a milder version)
1 lemon, peeled
3 tablespoons raw honey
Dash of turmeric
1 cup ice

Serves 1

Chocolate Shaker

1 frozen banana
1 cup almond milk (vanilla flavored)
1 tablespoon low-fat chocolate chips
    (find them at specialty food stores)
1 tablespoon cocoa powder
2 tablespoons peanut butter
1 teaspoon honey or agave

Serves 2

Note: For best results, stick a banana, peeled and wrapped in cellophane, in the freezer overnight. In the morning, throw the banana and the rest of the ingredients into a blender. Blend on high for about 30 seconds. This is crazy delicious, but keep in mind that it's quite filling. For a lighter version, lose the chocolate chips.

> ### PROTEIN POWDERS
>
> Protein helps to repair muscle tissue, which is important for muscle growth and strength. Lions and tigers get all the protein they need from their diet because they eat raw meat. Humans are often protein deficient because we tend to overcook our food, which destroys nutrients. That's why I recommend a daily protein supplement. Make sure to read the dosage instructions on the jar, and consult your doctor before taking any supplements. You'll find many different varieties and flavors in the health section of your local grocery store. Here are some of the most common types:
>
> - Whey protein. Whey takes 3 to 4 hours to digest, so it's a useful daytime supplement.
> - Casein protein. This is a good one for your evening meal, because it breaks down over about 7 hours. It's an anti-catabolic protein, meaning it counteracts the natural process of muscle breakdown. Basically it helps repair your muscles while you sleep.
> - Vegan protein. Great if you don't eat eggs, meat, or dairy. Examples include hemp, rice, soy, and spirulina protein.

JUICES

Back in Jamaica, my mother introduced me to the power and pleasure of juicing, which produces delicious drinks that also cleanse your body of toxins. Juicing takes a bit more prep and cleaning time than opening a store-bought can or a container, but the benefits to your health are worth it. You're guaranteed a drink with no added sweeteners, preservatives, or other harmful chemicals. Some other benefits of juicing include:

- Softer and clearer skin
- Improved immune system
- Weight loss
- Increased energy
- Elimination of waste
- Increased blood flow

Important guidelines:

- Make sure to thoroughly wash your fruits and vegetables before juicing them.
- Juicers extract liquid from your fruits and vegetables, leaving the fiber behind. You can always save the leftover fiber from juicing and use it as a flavoring for soups, salads, and other dishes.

- Juicers come in many shapes, styles, and price points. Choose the one that works for you and follow the manufacturer's operating instructions.
- Cut up your fruits and vegetables so they fit in the juicer.
- Drink your juice immediately after preparation.
- If you want to preserve your juice, you can do so for no more than 30 minutes by adding the juice of ½ lemon and refrigerating.

Power Supply

6 carrots
1 cored apple
1 cucumber
3 stalks celery

Serves 1

Iron Man

1 red beet
3 carrots
½ inch piece of ginger, peeled

Serves 1

Taste-Bud Enhancer

4 large slices pineapple
4 large slices watermelon
4 large slices cantaloupe

Serves 1

Caribbean Eye Opener

3 kiwis
1 cored apple
4 medium carrots
1 cup parsley

Serves 2

Note: Wrap the parsley around the carrots before you drop them in the juicer. You get more juice from the parsley if it's wrapped around the carrot—go figure.

Immune Station

3 stalks celery
1 cup kale
1 cup spinach
½ cup wheatgrass (tastes horrible, but is very good for you)
Juice of ½ lemon

Serves 1

Slimmer You

2 large pink grapefruits
½ cup diced pineapple
1-inch piece of ginger, peeled
½ lemon

Serves 1

Healthy Melody

2 cups cabbage
2 stalks celery
3 carrots

Serves 1

Vitamin C Madness

1 large pink grapefruit
2 kiwis
2 oranges

Serves 1

Sounds Nasty but Good for You

1 cup broccoli
½ cup green cabbage
2 cups spinach

Serves 1

Dracula's Dream

2 beetroots
Juice of 1 lemon

Serves 1

EGGS

My breakfast recipes are intended for cooks who have minimal time and experience in the kitchen and like to keep it that way. Don't skip breakfast—evidence shows that those who do slow down their metabolism and are prone to overeating later in the day.

Egg-cellent (Scrambled)

2 large eggs
2 egg whites
½ large yellow onion, finely chopped
1 clove garlic, finely chopped
1 teaspoon dried rosemary
1 teaspoon extra-virgin olive oil
Dash or two of sea salt

Crack the large eggs into a mixing bowl. Add the egg whites and whisk. Stir in the onion, garlic, and rosemary. Meanwhile, heat the olive oil in a medium-size frying pan. Pour the egg mixture into the pan and fold gently until the egg mixture can be peeled away from the pan (about 2 minutes). Add sea salt to taste and serve!

Serves 1

PERFECT HARD-BOILED EGGS

Don't be ashamed if you can't boil an egg properly. Not everyone knows how to do it right. This is my favorite method: In a small pot, cover the eggs with cold water and bring to a boil. Reduce the heat to low, cover the pan, and continue to simmer for 6 to 8 minutes. Remove the eggs from the hot water and put in a bowl with ice water for a minute or two, then peel. The shells will come off without sticking and you will have perfectly cooked hard-boiled eggs.

Egg on a Pita

1 hard-boiled egg, coarsely chopped
1 scallion, chopped
1 slice tomato, chopped and seeded
1 teaspoon finely chopped onion
1 teaspoon unsalted butter
½ pocket pita

Mix the egg, scallion, tomato, and onion in a small bowl. Spread the butter inside the pita, stuff in the egg mixture, and serve.

Serves 1

One Love Eggwich

1 whole wheat English muffin, toasted
1 teaspoon light mayo
1 lightly fried egg (over easy with a little extra-virgin olive oil)
1 slice tomato
2 thin slices avocado
Sea salt and pepper

Toast the English muffin and spread thinly with light mayo. Add the fried egg and layer on the tomato and avocado. Sprinkle with sea salt and pepper to taste and top with the other half of the muffin.

Serves 1

THE MAGIC OF FLAXSEED

I'm a big fan of flaxseed. It's a great source of fiber and omega-3, a natural fatty acid that has been shown to improve brain functioning, lower your risk of heart disease, and reduce the inflammation associated with rheumatoid arthritis and other common ailments. Flaxseed is widely available at specialty food stores and, increasingly, supermarkets. It comes ground or in whole seeds and has a pleasant nutty flavor. I usually add a couple of tablespoons to my smoothies, soups, and salads.

GRAINS

I Can't Believe This Is Oatmeal

1 cup rolled oats
½ banana, mashed
3 dashes of ground cinnamon
1 teaspoon flaxseed
2 cups almond milk
1 teaspoon organic peanut butter

Combine all ingredients in a saucepan and bring to a boil. Reduce the heat and simmer for about 6 minutes, or until the mixture thickens. If it gets too thick, add a little water until you get the desired consistency. If you have a little extra time, cover the pan after the oatmeal is fully cooked and let it rest for 10 minutes before serving. This produces a luxurious, creamy mixture that tastes like a dessert but is perfectly nutritious.

Serves 2

Cere-o's

1 bowl of your favorite high-fiber cereal. I love Kashi, but there are many choices in the cereal aisle of your local grocery store. Just don't get sidetracked by all that sugary nonsense. Skip any cereal with more than 25 grams of sugar per serving.

Serve with 1 cup of almond milk, 1 sliced banana, 2 dashes of grated nutmeg, and 1 teaspoon ground flaxseed.

Serves 1

Banana YUMcakes

Extra-virgin olive oil or unsalted butter for greasing the pan
2 cups whole wheat pancake mix
3 dashes of grated nutmeg
1⅓ cups cold water or almond milk
½ ripe banana, sliced
2 to 3 tablespoons chopped walnuts

Toppings (optional)

1 ripe banana, sliced (per batch)
2 teaspoons finely chopped walnuts (per batch)
1 teaspoon fat-free caramel topping (per pancake)

Heat a skillet or griddle over medium-high heat. Grease with olive oil or unsalted butter. In a medium mixing bowl, combine the pancake mix, nutmeg, and water or almond milk and whisk until smooth. The batter will be slightly thin. Stir in the banana and walnuts. **Note:** Do not overmix the batter. It will make the pancakes very tough.

For each pancake, pour slightly less than ¼ cup batter onto the hot greased skillet. Cook until bubbles break on the surface and the edges just begin to brown. Turn; cook about 1 minute more or until the bottoms come off the skillet effortlessly.

Serves 2

SANDWICHES

PB Wafflewich

2 whole-grain waffles
1½ tablespoons natural peanut butter
1 tablespoon natural honey
2 to 3 strawberries, sliced (replaces traditional jelly)
Pinch of ground cinnamon

This is a sinfully good, filling, yet healthy meal—and not just for breakfast! Toast the waffles until lightly browned. Spread the peanut butter and honey on one waffle, layer on the strawberries, and sprinkle them with cinnamon. Top with the second waffle, slice the sandwich in half, and devour. You'll never go back to the traditional PBJ sandwich again!

Serves 1

Life-Changing Avocado Cranberry Cheesewich

1 tablespoon ricotta cheese
2 slices whole wheat bread, toasted
½ tomato, sliced
½ avocado, sliced
1 teaspoon dried cranberries

Spread the ricotta on one toast slice. Layer on the tomato and avocado slices and cranberries. Top with the second slice of toast, slice your sandwich in half, and chow down.

Serves 1

Leftover Chicken Salad Sandwich

Whenever you have leftover chicken from one of my chicken dishes (starting on page 173) or a rotisserie bird that you don't know what to do with, turn it into a delectable lunch. Tomato and pickles give the sandwich a zesty homemade flair. If you want more intensity without adding calories, add a dash of sweet curry spice, a splash of apple cider vinegar, and a fresh herb such as dill, cilantro, or mint.

    1 cup diced leftover chicken breast
    ½ stalk celery, finely chopped
    1 tablespoon low-fat mayonnaise
    2 slices wheat bread (toasted or plain)
    ½ medium bell pepper, cut into 3-inch slices
    2 slices tomato
    4 slices from a small kosher pickle

Toss the chicken and celery with the mayo until lightly coated. Spoon the mixture onto one slice of bread, top with the pepper, tomato, and pickle slices, cover with the second slice of bread, and devour.

Serves 1

Veggie Power Wrap

You'll never miss the animal protein in this colorful, crunchy, heart-healthy wrap. If you like your wraps spicy, add a little adobo sauce or Tabasco to taste.

Note: Most of my recipes can be packed in watertight containers for lunch at work or on the go. The Veggie Power Wrap is an exception, as it can get a bit messy if jostled. I recommend eating it on the spot.

    1 cup canned red kidney beans, drained and rinsed
    1 teaspoon sea salt
    1 cup shredded cabbage
    1 cup baby spinach
    ½ onion, coarsely chopped
    1 bell pepper, coarsely chopped

1 yellow squash, coarsely chopped
1 teaspoon dried basil
3 whole wheat wraps
½ avocado, sliced (save the other half for later: wrap tightly in plastic and store in the fridge)
1 Roma tomato, coarsely chopped

Place the beans in a small saucepan, season with the salt, and cook covered over medium heat for 5 minutes. Remove from the heat and reserve.

Place the cabbage in ½ cup water in a saucepan with a tight-fitting lid. Bring the water to a boil, and steam the cabbage for 8 to 10 minutes. Then stir in the spinach, onion, pepper, squash, and basil, replace the lid, and steam for an additional 5 minutes. Allow the vegetables to cool—I like my wraps lukewarm.

Place a wrap on a flat surface. Spoon a third of the cabbage mixture evenly over 1 side of the wrap (nearest you). Spread a third of the beans over the cabbage mixture. Layer a third of the avocado and tomato over the beans. Fold the edge of the wrap over the ingredients, tuck in the sides, and roll the wrap tightly away from you. Repeat for the other 2 wraps.

Serves 3

Amazing Tuna Salad

This is my healthy, savory take on an American classic. For an extra zing, season with a pinch of salt and a dash of either vinegar or lemon juice.

1 (5-ounce) can tuna packed in water or oil
(*Note:* I prefer the taste of water-packed tuna, but some nutritionists are now saying that oil-packed tuna is healthier because the oil preserves the nutrients in the fish. Oil-packed tuna has a bit more fat, but either choice will provide a low-carbohydrate, high-protein boost to your diet.)
1 tablespoon finely chopped red onion
1 scallion, finely chopped
¼ teaspoon crushed dried peppers
1 teaspoon dried basil
1 tablespoon low-fat mayonnaise

Spoon the tuna into a small bowl. Mix in the onion, scallion, peppers, basil, and mayo. Serve on wheat crackers.

Serves 2

VEGETABLES

Pacific Stir-Fry Cabbage

Although I'm from Jamaica and I love Caribbean food, I'm also inspired by many other culinary traditions, including Asian cuisine. My take on the classic stir-fry makes it a colorful and fresh side for any dish.

    3 tablespoons extra-virgin olive oil
    1 whole green cabbage, shredded
    3 carrots, grated or shredded
    1 onion, chopped
    2 scallions, coarsely chopped
    2 cloves garlic, finely chopped
    1 head broccoli, coarsely chopped
    1 sweet pepper, chopped
    Dash of sea salt
    2 teaspoons apple cider vinegar
    Fresh or dried thyme, to taste
    Fresh or dried basil, to taste
    Fresh or dried oregano, to taste
    Cayenne pepper, to taste

Heat the oil in a wok or a deep sauté pan. Stir-fry all the ingredients at once, adding thyme, basil, oregano, and cayenne pepper to taste (a dash of cayenne is plenty if you are not used to spicy food). Add about ¼ cup water, enough to prevent the oil from burning and allow the vegetables to steam. Add more water, a splash at a time, as needed. Cook on medium heat for 30 minutes, stirring frequently. Serve with brown rice.

Serves 2

Stew Peas

When I was growing up in Jamaica, my mom's stew peas were one of my favorite dishes. Even now I get a smile on my face just thinking about them. Note that Scotch bonnet peppers are seasonal, so if your local store isn't carrying them, you can try using habañero, jalapeño, or serrano peppers. They are not interchangeable, but you need some kind of heat to make this dish really sing. Always be careful when chopping hot peppers such as these. Wear gloves and wash your hands if they come in contact with the seeds.

2 cups dried red peas, soaked in cold water overnight, or substitute canned kidney beans
2 cloves garlic, finely chopped
2 tablespoons dried thyme
3 scallions, coarsely chopped
1 large red onion, coarsely chopped
½ Scotch bonnet pepper, finely chopped
Sea salt and pepper

Put the peas, garlic, thyme, scallions, onion, and Scotch bonnet pepper in a saucepan, and add just enough water to cover. Cook over medium heat for about 20 minutes, until the mixture thickens. Season with sea salt and pepper to taste. Serve with 1 cup boiled jasmine rice.

Serves 2

Sweet and Sour Broccoli

This exotic but easy-to-make medley of vegetables makes broccoli look and taste glamorous. If you really want to live on the gastronomically wild side, serve it next to quinoa, couscous, or buckwheat groats.

2 carrots, grated
1 head broccoli, separated into spears
1 teaspoon extra-virgin olive oil
½ cup shiitake mushrooms, cleaned and coarsely chopped
4 cloves garlic, finely chopped
1 teaspoon sea salt
1 teaspoon honey or agave
Juice of 1 medium-size orange (or ½ cup orange juice)
Juice of 1 lemon
1 medium bell pepper, sliced into 3-inch pieces

Cook the grated carrots in 1 quart boiling water for 4 to 5 minutes. Drain the water and reserve the carrots.

Place the broccoli and ½ cup water in a large saucepan with a tight-fitting lid. Crank the burner to high and steam for 2 to 3 minutes, until the broccoli turns dark green. Turn off the flame and reserve.

Heat the olive oil in a small frying pan. Throw in the mushrooms, garlic, sea salt, and sweetener. Cook for 1 minute, stirring constantly.

Combine the carrots, broccoli, and mushrooms in a mixing bowl. Stir in the orange and lemon juices. Add the pepper and stir well so that the veggies are nicely coated. Serve with your choice of grains.

Serves 2

CHICKEN

Bull Bay Stew Chicken with Broccoli and Sweet Potato

In Jamaican cooking, a "stew" dish refers to protein simmered in gravy on the stovetop. My mom used to cook stew chicken when I was growing up in Bull Bay, Jamaica, and later in the South Bronx. When I was a kid I would watch her in the kitchen, feeling the love and joy that she always brought to cooking. And it tasted amazing!

1 small sweet potato, cubed (about 1 cup)
Kosher salt or sea salt
Extra-virgin olive oil
4-ounce chicken breast, cubed into bite-size pieces
Fresh or dried basil, to taste
Ground allspice, to taste
1 dash cayenne pepper
½ cup diced sweet pepper (any color)
½ onion, finely chopped
2 small carrots, finely chopped or grated
¾ cup water
1 teaspoon Gravy Master Seasoning and Browning Sauce, for color (*Note:* If you don't have Gravy Master, try 1 teaspoon soy sauce mixed with 1 teaspoon mirin [rice wine].)
1 cup steamed broccoli spears
½ small avocado, sliced

Preheat the oven to 425°F. Season the sweet potato with salt, place in an ovenproof dish in a single layer, drizzle with olive oil, and bake on the middle rack until soft, about 20 minutes. Flip occasionally to prevent sticking and burning.

Season the chicken with salt, basil, allspice, and cayenne pepper. In a preheated, oiled, nonstick cooking pan, quickly brown the chicken cubes on all sides over a medium flame.

Add the sweet pepper, onion, and carrots to the pan, stir-frying the mixture, gradually adding water to moisten and blend the flavors. Drizzle with the browning sauce, reduce the heat to low, and simmer over a low flame for about 12 minutes, stirring frequently, until the vegetables are soft and fragrant. Add more water, if needed, to the sauce.

To serve, place the stew at the center of the plate, and surround it with steamed broccoli, sweet potato, and avocado.

Serves 2

Spicy Salsa Chicken

This dish is easy to make and tastes even better when reheated. If you are not using cheese, you can prepare it in advance and enjoy it straight out of the refrigerator. Use salt at your discretion—some taco seasoning mixes are saltier than others, so you be the judge.

    2 skinless, boneless chicken breast halves
    1 tablespoon plus 1 teaspoon liquid taco seasoning mix (many varieties are available in grocery
        stores; pick your favorite)
    1 teaspoon salt, optional
    1 small onion, chopped
    2 teaspoons dried parsley
    1 teaspoon rosemary
    ⅔ cup of your favorite spicy salsa
    1 cup shredded cheddar cheese

Preheat the oven to 400°F. Place the chicken breasts in an oven-safe dish. Spread the taco seasoning mix evenly over the chicken, then sprinkle the salt (if using), onion, parsley, and rosemary on top. Pour the salsa over the chicken and spread it evenly with the back of a spoon. Bake in the center of the oven for 20 to 22 minutes. Remove, sprinkle the cheese on top, and put it back in the oven for another 5 minutes. Serve with 1 cup brown rice or quinoa.

Serves 2

Island Bok Choy with Chicken

The colorful medley of vegetables and chicken make this a complete meal nutritionally, but it is also a great vegetarian side dish if you want to omit the chicken. It is delicious served hot or cold.

Note: For tastier chicken, marinate the breast for 30 minutes before baking in a mixture of your favorite West Indian hot sauce, chopped garlic, salt, pepper, lime juice, and agave. Marinating will also yield nicely caramelized meat as it bakes.

3 ounces chicken breast, cubed
Salt and black pepper, to taste
2 to 3 bunches baby bok choy, or 1 bunch regular bok choy, coarsely chopped
1 red bell pepper, coarsely chopped
1 large onion, coarsely chopped
3 cloves garlic, finely chopped
1 head broccoli, cut into spears
1 teaspoon dried, crushed red peppers
1 teaspoon dried thyme, or 1 tablespoon fresh thyme leaves
3 stalks celery, finely chopped
2 cups baby spinach

Preheat the oven to 400°F. Season the chicken with salt and pepper (or marinate as above) and bake the chicken in an ovenproof dish for 15 minutes, until the juices that the chicken cubes release turn white. Remove from the oven and reserve.

Heat ½ cup salted water in a large saucepan. Throw in the bok choy, bell pepper, onion, garlic, broccoli, crushed red pepper, thyme, and celery. Cover and steam over medium heat until the bok choy turns dark green (about 5 minutes).

Add the spinach to the bok choy mixture. Simmer for another 5 minutes. Combine the vegetables with the chicken and let the mixture stand, covered, for another 5 minutes to absorb flavors. Serve with 1 baked red potato, or 1 cup brown rice or quinoa.

Serves 2

OMG! Chicken Couscous Salad

This easy-to-make salad is rich in flavor and gets better over time. It is naturally sweet, but if you like your salads on the acidic, spicy side, at the end balance it out with a splash of lemon juice, a dash of salt and pepper, and a tablespoon of apple cider.

For the Chicken:

4- to 5-ounce chicken breast, cubed
½ teaspoon salt

Preheat the oven to 400°F. Bake the cubed chicken breast, lightly salted, in an oven-safe dish for 15 minutes. Remove from the oven and reserve.

Note: Bake an extra 4 or 5 ounces of chicken breast and reserve for a Leftover Chicken Salad Sandwich (page 169).

For the Salad Dressing:

3 tablespoons balsamic vinegar
1 cup fresh-squeezed orange juice
2 teaspoons honey or agave
¼ cup extra-virgin olive oil

Combine the vinegar, orange juice, and sweetener in a mixing bowl. Whisk in the olive oil in a steady steam so it emulsifies evenly. Reserve.

For the Salad:

1 cup whole wheat couscous
1 bell pepper, diced
1 cucumber, diced
1 tomato, diced and seeded
3-inch piece of ginger, grated
1 handful of baby spinach
1 onion, coarsely chopped
1 green apple, chopped
2 cloves garlic, finely chopped
1 carrot, shredded
¼ cup crushed or slivered almonds

Cook the couscous according to the instructions on the box and allow to cool. Add the bell pepper, cucumber, tomato, ginger, spinach, onion, apple, garlic, carrot, and almonds. Stir until the ingredients are well mixed. Add the chicken breast and dressing and mix thoroughly. Let the salad rest for 10 to 15 minutes to absorb flavors before serving.

Serves 2 to 4

SEAFOOD

Yardie Brown Stew Fish with Steamed Cabbage

"Yard" is Jamaican slang for back home, and we Jamaicans call ourselves "yardies". A stew may not be a conventional lunch choice in America, but yardies crave it for lunch, especially on a beautiful sunny day.

8-ounce red snapper fillet, skin on (a 2½-pound fish will yield about 2 8-ounce fillets)
Dash of cayenne pepper
Dried thyme, to taste
Dried basil, to taste
Sea salt, to taste
1 tablespoon extra-virgin olive oil
2 carrots, finely chopped
½ onion, finely chopped
1 clove garlic, diced or mashed
1 teaspoon Gravy Master Browning Sauce
1 cup diced fresh green cabbage
Juice of 1 lime (optional)
2 scallions, green and white parts, chopped (optional)

Preheat a large frying pan. Season the fish with cayenne pepper, thyme, basil, and sea salt. Fry the fish, skin side up, in the olive oil for 2 minutes. Remove the fish and reserve, covered. Add the carrots, onion, garlic, and browning sauce to the pan and stir-fry for 5 minutes, until the vegetables caramelize. Add water, a teaspoon or so at a time, to loosen up the vegetables and prevent burning. Lower the heat, return the fish to the pan, and cook skin side down, covered, for another 4 to 6 minutes. Meanwhile, steam the cabbage in ½ cup boiling water in a tightly covered saucepan for about 5 minutes. To serve the dish, place the fish over the cabbage, and top it with the vegetable mixture. Top with lime juice and scallions (if using).

Serves 1

Curry Shrimp

This is a gourmet-style light meal you don't have to be a fancy chef to prepare. If you want to kick up the flavor a notch, you can finish by adding grated ginger, chopped cilantro, and a squeeze of lime juice.

1 medium onion, finely chopped
2 tablespoons extra-virgin olive oil
1 teaspoon sea salt
2 scallions, chopped
1 red bell pepper, cut into 3-inch slices
2 cloves garlic, finely chopped
2 teaspoons curry powder
1 sprig fresh thyme

½ cup water
1 pound jumbo shrimp, shelled and deveined
2 tablespoons unsweetened coconut milk

In a thick-bottomed pot, preferably a Dutch oven, sauté the onion in the olive oil and a dash of salt until it starts caramelizing, about 12 minutes, stirring constantly. Add the scallions, pepper, garlic, curry powder, and thyme and continue sautéing for another 5 to 8 minutes. Add the water and shrimp, bring to a boil, and reduce the heat to low. When the shrimp is cooked thoroughly (it turns pink and curls into an almost perfect circle), slowly pour the coconut milk into the curry, stirring and simmering gently for another 2 minutes. Turn off the heat and adjust the seasoning if necessary. Inhale the aroma and imagine an exotic vacation at sea. Serve with 1 cup brown rice.

Serves 2 to 4

Salmon with Honey Glaze

This simple weeknight dinner is filling and keeps fresh overnight. Save the leftovers, if any, for lunch the next day. If you want a guilt-free side of carbs, serve this dish with a side of potatoes smashed with a couple of drops of olive oil, salt, pepper, and your choice of fresh green herbs.

4 (3-ounce) wild sockeye salmon steaks, skin on
Sea salt and pepper
1 red onion, coarsely chopped
2 tablespoons dried thyme
1 large tomato, coarsely chopped
2 cloves garlic, finely chopped
1 large red bell pepper, coarsely chopped
1 tablespoon honey diluted with juice of ½ orange or 1 lemon

Preheat the oven to 400°F. Season the salmon steaks with salt and pepper, and place them in an oven-safe dish, skin side down. Spread the onion, thyme, tomato, garlic, and pepper around the salmon. Bake in the center of the oven for 10 minutes. Remove from the oven, but leave the oven on. Using a brush, spread the honey glaze over the steaks and return them to the oven for an additional 2 minutes. Remove from the oven and allow to cool for several minutes before serving. Debone the steaks if you wish, and serve with ½ cup of smashed red potatoes per serving, if using.

Serves 2 to 4

Shrimp, Rice, and Beans Delight

This is a great meal for when you're dead tired. I can whip this up in my sleep.

    2 cups brown rice
    1 cup canned black beans, drained and rinsed
    1 can whole kernel sweet corn (*no cream*)
    2 carrots, diced
    1 small onion, finely chopped
    2 scallions, finely chopped
    1 teaspoon dried basil
    1 teaspoon dried cilantro
    1 teaspoon dried thyme
    2 stalks celery, finely chopped
    1 pound baby shrimp, peeled and deveined

Bring 4 cups of water to a boil in a large saucepan with a tight-fitting lid. Throw in the brown rice, cover the pan with the lid, and cook over medium heat for 25 to 30 minutes, or until all the water is absorbed and the rice grains are soft.

    Note: If the rice dries out too fast, add a bit more water.

In another saucepan, bring 1 cup of water to a boil. Throw in the beans, corn, carrots, onion, scallions, basil, cilantro, thyme, and celery. Cover and cook for about 5 minutes over medium heat. After 5 minutes, add the shrimp and cook for another 3 to 5 minutes, until the shrimp fold up and turn pink. Remove from the flame and combine the shrimp mixture with the rice. Enjoy!

Serves 4 to 6

SOUPS

Energy Soup

This is a hearty rustic soup of root and green vegetables thickened with beans. It tastes too good to be vegetarian. For an elegant presentation, puree with a handheld blender and serve with a drizzle of olive oil, a sprinkling of fresh thyme leaves, ½ finely chopped, seeded jalapeño pepper, and lemon zest on top. You'll have about 15 servings, so freeze the remainder for later use.

    2 turnips, peeled and coarsely chopped
    3 carrots, peeled and sliced
    1 onion, coarsely chopped

2 red potatoes, cubed

2 batata yams, peeled and cubed

1 cup red kidney beans, canned or fresh

Sea salt

1 head broccoli, split into spears

2 cloves garlic, finely chopped

3 stalks celery, coarsely chopped

2 sprigs thyme

2 chayotes, peeled and cubed

Bring the turnips, carrots, onion, potatoes, yams, and kidney beans to a boil in a large saucepan filled with 2 quarts of salted water. Reduce the heat and throw in the broccoli, garlic, celery, thyme, and chayotes and cook for about 15 minutes over medium-high heat, until the soup thickens and all the vegetables are soft. Adjust the seasonings if desired and serve!

Serves 12 to 15

Rasta Peas Soup

Jamaicans who follow the Rastafarian faith believe in eating only vegetarian food. Some of my relatives are Rastas, and I've always been inspired by their earthy lifestyle. Everything Rastas eat comes from the ground—they call it "Ital" food. Here's my Ital version of a classic Jamaican dish, pea soup. You'll have enough soup for about 15 servings, so share it with your family and friends or freeze for later use.

1-pound bag dried red peas, soaked in water for 24 hours and rinsed (If time is short, you can substitute canned peas or kidney beans, drained and rinsed to remove salt.)

2 chayotes (also called chochos), peeled, seeded, and chopped into 1-inch chunks (Substitute turnips if you can't find chayotes.)

1½ cups diced pumpkin or butternut squash (see note)

6 medium carrots, chopped

1 large sweet onion, chopped

3 red potatoes, chopped

4 stalks celery, chopped

Dash of sea salt

3 pinches of dried thyme

2 tablespoons chopped scallions (approximately 3 stalks, trimmed and peeled)

Note: If using pumpkin, make sure to clean it properly: Cut it in half and scoop out all the seeds and fiber from the center of each half.

Place the peas, chayotes, pumpkin, carrots, onion, potatoes, and celery in a large pot. Cover with double the amount of water. Bring to a boil, reduce the heat to medium, and continue simmering for 20 minutes.

Add the sea salt, thyme, and scallions. Simmer for 5 more minutes, and then serve.

Serves 12 to 15

Trenchtown Lentil Soup

Jamaicans love lentil soup. I cook mine in water, but if you want even more flavor, try it with vegetable broth. Cook with a bay leaf for smokier flavor. This is a rustic, chunky soup that's colorful and vibrant in texture. If you want a more elegant, formal presentation, puree the soup, after it cools, with a handheld blender and serve it with a sprinkle of freshly chopped parsley.

1 teaspoon extra-virgin olive oil
1 medium onion, minced
2 carrots, sliced
Pinch of cayenne pepper
1 teaspoon dried thyme
1 teaspoon dried parsley
1 cup dried lentils, rinsed
2 quarts water or vegetable broth
1 bay leaf, optional
1 red potato, coarsely chopped
1 cup finely chopped kale
1 tomato, coarsely chopped
Sea salt, to taste

Heat the olive oil in a thick-bottomed soup pot. Sauté the onion and carrots for 15 minutes, until the vegetables caramelize, stirring frequently with a wooden spoon. Add the pepper, thyme, parsley, and lentils and stir.

Add the water, bay leaf (if using), and potato and bring to a boil. Add the kale and tomato, lower the heat, and simmer for another 20 minutes, until all the vegetables are soft. Salt to taste and you are done!

Serves 6 to 8

DESSERTS

Like all eaters, I have my philosophy about dessert. It's simple enough: Deprivation never works, so if you need sugar, you are going to have to satisfy your craving somehow. Just because you are getting in shape doesn't mean sucking all the joy out of eating. My desserts are flourless, rely on fruit and other earthy goodness, permit some indulgence in better-quality dairy products, and are simple to make.

Fresh Fruit with Yogurt

4 tablespoons Greek yogurt
1 small mango, sliced
4 strawberries, sliced
(Or substitute any combination of your favorite fruits)

If you are feeling feisty, drizzle with a little honey and sprinkle with chopped walnuts.

Serves 1

Fresh Fruit Kabob with Chocolate Fondue

1 cup dark chocolate chips
1 tablespoon almond milk
2 bananas, sliced
12 strawberries, sliced

Melt the chocolate chips in a double boiler with the almond milk, stirring constantly to make sure the chocolate doesn't burn. Pour the melted chocolate into a fondue pot over a low flame. Slice the bananas and strawberries and place on a platter with wood skewers. Using the skewers, dip the fruit into the melted chocolate and chow down. (Make sure the chocolate isn't too hot!) Invite some friends to join you. Have plenty of napkins on hand.

Serves 4

Stuffed Caramelized Apples

If you want your dessert to come out of the oven dressed to kill, try this simple option, inspired by a clean-cut and delicious dessert that once appeared on the menu of the Caribbean-inspired restaurant A on the Upper West Side of Manhattan.

1 green apple
2 tablespoons soft goat cheese
2 teaspoons honey
½ teaspoon fresh thyme leaves
1 dash ground cinnamon
1 teaspoon slivered almonds

Preheat the oven to 400°F. Split and core the apple. Mash the goat cheese with a drizzle of honey and thyme leaves. Stuff the apple cavities with the cheese mixture. Wrap the apple halves in heavy-duty foil without letting the foil make contact with the apple flesh or the cheese. Bake on a cookie sheet for 15 to 20 minutes, checking to make sure the apple halves are soft but don't fall apart. Remove from the oven and allow to cool slightly. Sprinkle with cinnamon, drizzle with the remaining honey, top with almonds, and dig in. This is a pretty hearty dessert, so split it with a loved one!

Serves 2

Chocolate Pudding

1 avocado, peeled and pitted
2 tablespoons cocoa powder
¼ cup water
3 dried dates, pitted
Dash of vanilla

Mix all the ingredients together in your blender, and please feel free to add more cocoa to taste. Use more water for a thinner pudding, and less water if you like it thicker.

Serves 2

Jamaica's Finest Fruit Salad

1 grapefruit, peeled, sectioned, and sliced
1 orange, peeled, sectioned, and sliced
1 ripe mango, peeled and sliced
3 tablespoons evaporated milk
2 dashes of grated nutmeg
2 dashes of ground cinnamon
1 scoop vanilla-flavored protein powder (Choose your favorite protein supplement—see box, page 162)
1 tablespoon honey or agave

Throw the grapefruit, orange, and mango in a bowl. Add the evaporated milk, nutmeg, cinnamon, protein powder, and honey. Stir until the fruit is evenly coated, and serve.

Serves 2

SNACKS

Tea and Almonds

1 handful of raw almonds
1 cup prepared peppermint tea

I also love dandelion tea, along with alfalfa, peppermint, spearmint, chamomile, lemon, and ginger tea. Cerasee tea from Jamaica is also delicious, and increasingly available in groceries in "foreign," which is the Jamaican term for North America.

Fruit Flava

6 strawberries, sliced
½ cup raspberries
½ cup blueberries

Throw the berries in a bowl and eat!

PB&A

1 apple, sliced
2 tablespoons natural peanut butter

Spread the peanut butter on the apple slices and enjoy!

APPENDIXES

APPENDIX A

Donovan's 3-Day Juice Cleanse

Remember, nutrition is 80 percent of fitness. Here's a 3-day cleanse that will optimize your metabolism for its main job, which is to burn calories. The goal is to cut out all refined sugars and animal products. You will consume nothing but raw vegetables, fruits, nuts, and juices.

This will be challenging for most, but you must follow the program if you are serious about losing weight and getting healthier. Please consult with your physician before you take part in this section of the program.

Here are four simple questions that will help you gauge your readiness to take on this challenge:

- Do you feel your health could be better?
- Are you tired of being overweight?
- Are you tired of feeling tired all the time?
- Are you afraid of dying young?

If you answered yes to any of these questions, you are more than ready to get started. If you are allergic to anything on the list, please substitute other foods from the same category. Drink at least 16 ounces of water with every meal and snack. Be sure to keep a log of your meals and workouts. Don't skip a day or a meal!

I recommend you do most of this cleanse over a weekend when you have time to stay home and relax. If you find yourself struggling to complete the cleanse, then I suggest that you just take your time and go day by day. Don't let yourself down by quitting. I need you to fight for what's right, and that is your life. Stay focused and be strong.

Caution: As your body begins to excrete toxins, you may experience withdrawal symptoms such as acne, headaches, insomnia, sore muscles, and fatigue. If you are a coffee drinker, you may experience these symptoms more intensely. Your body is accustomed to its routine. When you change that routine, your body will react in ways that may seem unnatural. Please allow your body to go through its process.

MEALS (ALL 3 DAYS)

Just like it's important to give your muscles time to recuperate after a workout, it's important to give your intestines a break every now and then. Here's a simple yet nutritious menu for your cleanse.

Breakfast

1 glass room-temperature water with the juice of ½ lemon
1 cup alfalfa tea, or your favorite herbal tea
Protein Power Hit smoothie (recipe on page 159)

Morning Snack

¼ cup raw or roasted almonds

Lunch

Power Supply juice (recipe on page 163)

Afternoon Snack

1 sliced apple spread with natural peanut butter

Dinner

1 bowl Trenchtown Lentil Soup (recipe on page 181)

Late-Night Snack

Immune Station juice (recipe on page 164)

APPENDIX B

Pantry List

If you want to break the fat cycle, shred your body, and feel as good as you will look, start by breaking some bad habits and establishing new, good ones. Begin by reviewing the contents of your pantry and refrigerator. Eliminate fatty, processed, unnatural food imitations that bring your mood down and your body weight up. Then restock the pantry and the refrigerator with items that will make this program enjoyable and hassle-free for you.

I have prepared a bulletproof fat-burning shopping list that will add zest and flavor to your diet. Remember, the way you eat will determine the way you look. If you eat lots of fatty foods, then you will be fat. If you eat clean and lean, then you will be lean, slim, and sexy.

Note: Always keep your pantry fully stocked. Never allow yourself to run low on these items or you'll be tempted by your old standbys. Your metabolism has to stay fully charged in order for this program to work at maximum capacity. *Let's go shopping!*

Beverages

Coffee beans, organic	Lemonade (homemade)
Iced tea, unsweetened or sweetened	Tea, herbal (peppermint, dandelion root, alfalfa, green, ginger)

Freezer

Chicken, organic	Steak, lean, grass-fed
Fruits, frozen	Turkey, organic
Ice cream, low-fat	Vegetables, frozen
Salmon, wild, or any other fatty fish	

Fruits

Apples	Oranges
Bananas	Peaches
Blackberries	Pineapples
Blueberries	Plums
Cantaloupe	Pomegranates
Grapefruit	Raspberries
Honeydew melon	Strawberries
Kiwis	Tangerines
Lemons/limes	Watermelon
Mangos	

Grains and Seeds

Brown rice	Flaxseed
Buckwheat	Quinoa
Bulgur	Steel-cut oats
Couscous	

Herbs and Spices

Basil, fresh or dried	Nutmeg, grated
Black pepper, ground	Onions
Cilantro, fresh or dried	Oregano, dried
Cinnamon, ground	Parsley, dried
Curry powder	Rosemary, fresh or dried
Garlic, fresh	Sea salt
Ginger, fresh	Thyme, fresh or dried
Mint, fresh	Turmeric

Nuts

Almonds	Pecans
Brazil nuts	Pistachios
Cedar nuts	Walnuts
Hazelnuts	

Oils

Coconut oil	Flaxseed oil
	Olive oil, extra-virgin

Pantry

Agave	Honey, organic
Balsamic vinegar	Kidney beans, canned
Brown sugar	Nut butters
Cereal, high-fiber	Pasta, wheat
Cereal, whole-grain	Sardines, canned
Corn, canned	Soups, low-fat, low-sodium, canned
Flour, wheat	Tuna in oil or water

Refrigerator

Cheese (Avoid processed options. I love natural cheddar and mozzarella, but there are hundreds of delicious artisanal cheeses on the market.)	Eggs Lemon juice Water, distilled or spring
Cottage cheese, low-fat	Yogurt, Greek

Slim Snacks

Cookies, low-sugar	Sherbet
Dried fruits	Strawberries (or other fruit) dipped in dark or milk chocolate
Frozen grapes	Trail mix
Ice cream, low-fat, with fresh fruits	Tuna with wheat crackers
Peanut butter and banana on whole wheat bread	Veggie chips
Pudding, sugar-free or fat-free	Wheat crackers with low-fat cheese
Rice cakes	

Vegetables

Asparagus	Kale
Avocados	Lettuce (iceberg, romaine, or Boston)
Beets	Onions
Bell peppers (green, red, yellow, and orange)	Red potatoes
Broccoli	Spinach
Cabbage	Squash, summer and winter
Carrots	Sweet potatoes
Celery	Tomatoes
Chayotes	Turnips
Cucumbers	Yams
Eggplant	Zucchini, yellow

APPENDIX C

Stretches

It's vital that you warm up and stretch before and after every workout. For example, warm up with 30 seconds of jumping jacks and then do the stretches below. Stretching releases stress and reduces the risk of injury to your muscles and joints. It also helps to increase your flexibility and range of motion. *Never forget to stretch!*

Here's a basic stretching regime that you should follow before and after every workout. Hold every stretch for about 20 seconds, and keep breathing throughout the stretch. Note: Stretching is not supposed to be painful, and it's quite easy to injure yourself by over-stretching. For each stretch, find that range where you are slightly uncomfortable but not in pain.

CROSSOVER HAMSTRING

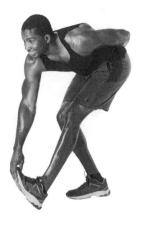

LATS AND SHOULDERS

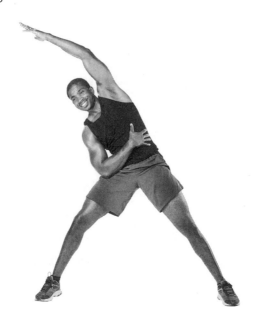

HAMSTRINGS, LATS, AND SHOULDERS

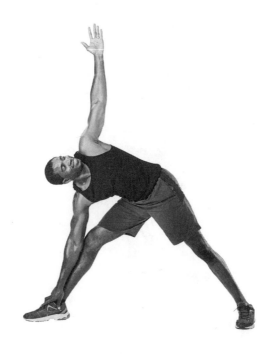

LATS AND HAMSTRINGS

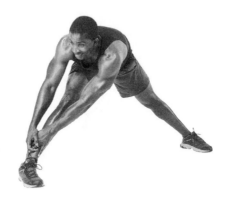

GROIN

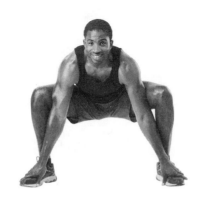

FOREARMS

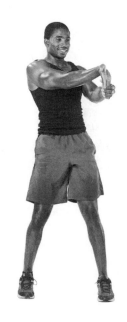

SHOULDERS

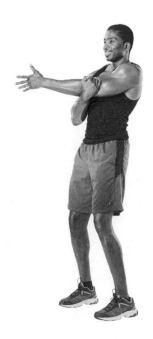

TRICEPS AND SHOULDERS

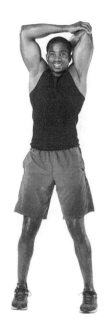

THIGHS (QUADRICEPS)

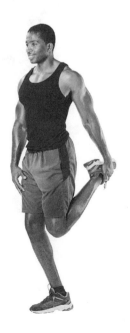

ADDUCTORS

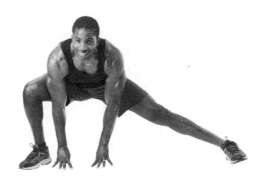

SPINE

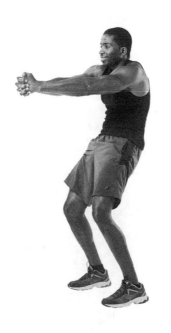

APPENDIX D

Sneak-Attack Workouts

Here are some alternate workouts that you can do on your rest days or whenever you feel like sneaking in a little extra exercise.

LOWER MY REPS

This is a very fast yet effective workout that will get your body warmed up from head to toe. Although it is fast, it is a butt kicker.

30 jumping jacks
30 push-ups (standard or from the knees)
30 sit-ups

Complete the moves back to back, and then repeat by dropping your reps down by increments of 5. For example: do 30 reps of each, then 25 of each, then 20, then 15, then 10, then 5.

STAIR RUNS

This is one of my favorite things to do when I travel or if I am not in the mood to go the gym. It will make you sweat like you just ran a 10K.

Run or walk up and down the stairs for 10 minutes as fast as you can.

Do 10 alternating knees every time you get to the bottom of the stairs: Stand with your feet parallel and shoulder width apart, knees soft, hands in fighting position. Bring your left leg up as high as you can, toes pointing to the floor. Repeat, alternating knees.

BLACK BELT SEQUENCE

This drill is designed to get your blood pumping and your joints loose. You muscles will burn and your heart rate will go through the roof. Oh yeah! You will burn some serious calories.

50 alternating front kicks
50 alternating knees
50 alternating straight punches
50 alternating uppercuts
50 crunches

Here is the fun part. Repeat this entire thing again. This time I want you to drop the reps down by 10. Keep doing this after the completion of the entire sequence (for example: do 50 reps of each, then 40 of each, then 30, then 20, then 10). Let's go, black belt!

GET YOUR BUTT OUTSIDE

Get outside and get some fresh air. I know this sounds too good to be true, and it is. I actually want you to walk/jog/run for a total of 1½ miles. Make sure to get your heart rate up.

APPENDIX E

Glossary

Aerobic exercise: With oxygen (for example, swimming, jumping rope, or jogging long distance).

Agility: The ability to change direction as fast as possible while in motion without losing acceleration.

Anaerobic exercise: With little or no oxygen (for example, lifting weights or sprinting).

Atrophy: Loss of muscle mass.

Calisthenics: Exercises that use your own body weight as resistance (for example, push-ups, pull-ups, and dips).

Explosive: Using maximum force in a very short period of time (for example, bench-pressing a certain amount of weight as fast as possible).

Hypertrophy: Increase of muscle mass gained from the strength-training phase of this program.

Power: How fast you can move a specific weight load away from your body, such as when doing a seated shoulder press.

Quickness: The ability to change direction on command, such as the blow of a whistle or the snap of a finger.

Speed: How fast you can get from one point to the next.

Strength: The number of times you can complete a specific move before fatigue sets in.

APPENDIX F

Additional Resources

Books

The Earth Diet, by Liana Werner-Gray
The Eat-Clean Diet, by Tosca Reno
Fuel for the Body, by Lynnette Marie
The Holy Bible
The Holy Quran
The Power of Focus, by Jack Canfield, Mark Victor Hansen, and Les Hewitt
Swim with the Sharks without Being Eaten Alive, by Harvey Mackay

Websites

www.doctoroz.com
www.healthcorps.org
www.projectslimdown.com
www.sharecare.com
www.webmd.com

APPENDIX G

The No Excuses Oath

I value your health just like I value my family's health. No offense to my friend Dr. Oz, but I want people like him to make less money from doing heart surgery. I'm doing my part, and I want you to do your part by vowing to live a healthier life. Repeat after me:

- *I solemnly swear to never bring harm to myself by introducing poison into my mind, spirit, or body.*
- *I will always be true to myself.*
- *I will allow nothing to disturb my peace.*
- *I will fight for what is right and never lose a battle to lack of will or determination.*
- *It is my right to live a life of joy and happiness with no prejudice to man, woman, or child.*
- *I will train my mind and body as hard as I can without bringing harm to myself or anyone else around me.*
- *I will eat lots of vegetables and fruits and cut down on the processed foods.*
- *I will be accountable for my own actions and blame no one else for my mistakes.*
- *I am the strongest, the most courageous, and the most respectful person you will meet.*
- *This is my life and I absolutely love who I am, but I understand that change is for the better.*

I want you to memorize this oath and say it to yourself every morning when you wake up. This will help you to break free from negativity and concentrate on the most important thing in your life: *you.*

ACKNOWLEDGMENTS

When I first decided to write this book, I had no idea where to start. I just got on my computer and started typing. I had a story to tell but I wasn't sure how to tell it. This is where my co-author Richard McGill Murphy came in. Richard helped me create a nice flow to my book by learning and understanding my style of speaking. He helped me to fill in the blanks, use what was needed, and lose what was not. Though I had full control, Richard gave suggestions that made perfect sense, and that's a great relationship. He also kept me on track and pushed me to keep going. Richard is the first person I would call if the opportunity came to write another book.

Richard and I both want to thank our peerless agent, Steve Hanselman, who saw the potential in this project very early and helped us navigate the publishing process with aplomb. We are also very grateful to the talented publishing team at Hachette Books, especially Mauro DiPreta, Stacy Creamer, Betsy Hulsebosch, Michelle Aielli, Melanie Gold, Cassie Mandel, Lauren Hummel, Eileen Chetti, Lori Paximadis, and the team at Jouve North America.

Julia Serebrinsky is a brilliant food and recipe editor who tested every recipe in this book, improved many of the dishes, and translated all my "little of this, dash of that" directions into recipes that readers can actually follow.

Lisa and Mehmet Oz are loyal friends and inspiring mentors who supported this book from the very beginning.

Eddie Berman is a gifted photographer who shot all the exercise pictures at his studio in Stamford, Connecticut. Thanks also to our beautiful and hardworking exercise models: Jeimy Bueno Canosa, Jason Kapowitz, Tina Kramer, Tricia Nisenson, and Cynthia Ramirez.

Peace and respect to all my Bronx brothers and sisters, especially George Bacot, Grementhia Flournoy, Danazsa Jones, Ronand Mainor, Grandmaster Melle Mel, and Daniel Robinson.

Heartfelt thanks to all my clients, especially Alex Cohen, Shirleen Dubuque, Kim Gilhool, John H. McClutchy Jr., Tricia Rosen, Joe Scarborough, and Laura Seely.

Finally, thanks and love to my family: Velma Harbour, Vincent Green, Ayana Green, Robert J. Little, Carmen Myers, Donovan Green Jr., Dorian Green, and Delani Green. This book is for you.

INDEX

reading, 136
refined sugar, 47–48
resilience, 30–31
resistance training. *See also* strength building
  butt and leg workout, 104–9, 127, 129
  calorie consumption, 113
  described, 103
rest days, 199–200
Rosen, Tricia, 61–62

S

SAD. *See* Standard American Diet
salad dressings, 88
salt, 100
sandwiches, 168–70
saving money, 101
scales, bathroom, xii, 54
schedule, exercise, 50
seafood recipes, 176–79
seated exercises, 73–101
sleep, 52–53, 66
Smith, Shoshana, xi–xii
smoothies, 157–61
snacks, 102, 184
soda, 96
soluble fiber, 51
soreness, 155
soups, 179–81
spices, 100
spiritual fitness, 34–37
stamina building
  interval training, 149–52
  punching and kicking exercises, 143–48
  seated exercises, 96–99, 102

Standard American Diet (SAD), 45
Starks, John, 24
Stevenson High School, 21
Stewart, Glen, 22
Stewart, Stepp, 24
strength building. *See also* resistance training
  benefits of, 63
  butt and leg exercises, 137–43
  core exercises, 124–27, 131–36
  importance of, 103
  interval training, 149–52
  kicking exercises, 131–36, 143–48
  muscle building, 128
  myths about, 110, 113, 128
  punching exercises, 143–48
  seated exercises, 73–88, 100, 101
  upper body exercises, 110–16, 128, 139–43
  yoga, 117–24, 129
stretches, 193–98
success, fear of, 6–7
sugar, refined, 47–48, 117
supermarkets, 48–49, 124
S.W.A.T. Team, 21
sweating, 101
sweeteners, 143

T

teasing, 19–20
technology, 13
Think phase, 70–102
Timberlake, Justin, 16
time, lack of, 13, 16–17
to-do lists, 85
trans fats, 136

U

UN Food and Agriculture Organization, 45
United Health Foundation, 11
universe, balanced, 35
University of Copenhagen, 60
upper body exercises, 110–16, 128, 139–43

V

vegetables, 85, 171–73
visualization exercises, 110, 139
vitamins, 51–52, 101
vocabulary, 124
volunteering, 130

W

walking, 100
warm-ups, 85
water intake, 50–51, 66, 72, 129, 152
weight lifting. *See* strength building
weight loss
  body mass index, 53
  calorie consumption, 46
  diet guidelines, 47–53
  exercise time, 60
  fad diets, 58, 59
  muscle *versus* fat, 155
  rate of, 11, 69
Wellness Tripod, 11, 12
willpower, 42–43
work relationships, 143

Y

yoga, 30, 117–24